Type 2 Diabetes Cookbook
for the Newly Diagnosed

Make food your ally

The complete guide to managing prediabetes and type 2 diabetes with fantastic easy-to-prepare healthy recipes for healthy living.

By
Rachel Rodriguez

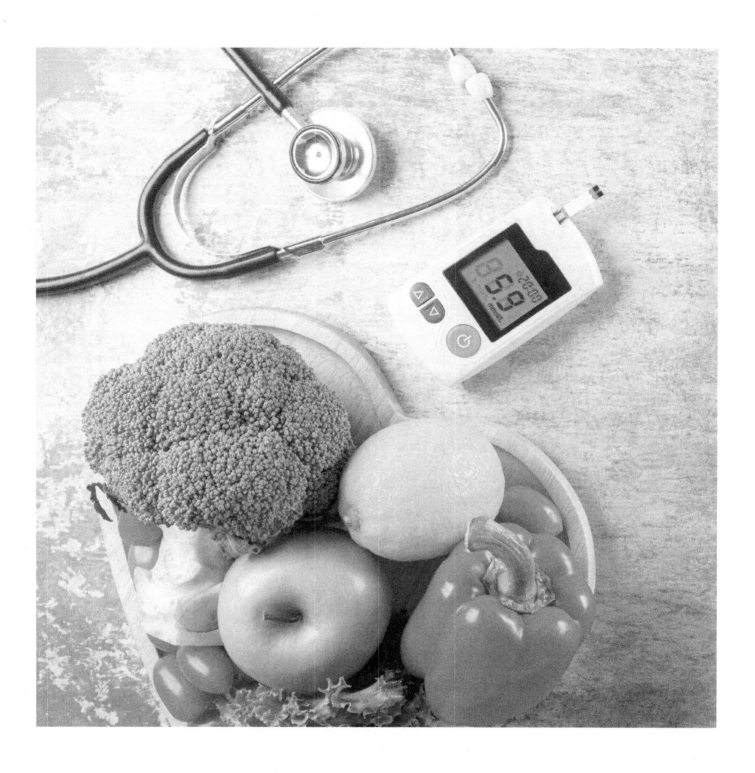

Table of Contents

CHAPTER 12: POULTRY RECIPES..108

CHAPTER 13: SEAFOOD RECIPES 117

CHAPTER 14: MEAT RECIPES 125

CHAPTER 15: SNACK RECIPES 133

Introduction

If you've got diagnosed with type 2 diabetes, one of the first things you might be concerned about is your diet. You'll almost certainly be bombarded with what seems like an endless stream of new assignments. With medical appointments, taking medicine, quitting smoking, becoming more sociable, and eating a balanced, nutritional diet, may all seem so overwhelming and difficult. With so much to absorb at once and all the misunderstandings about diabetes and diet that you'll almost certainly hear, it may be difficult to know what to do.

First and foremost, you should understand that there is no such thing as a particular diet for type 2 diabetes. There are no two diabetics who are exactly alike. As a result, just as there is no one-size-fits-all diet for diabetics, there is no one-size-fits-all diet for diabetics.

People with type 2 diabetes used to be sent home with a list of foods they weren't permitted to eat after their diagnosis or even told to cut out sugar. However, we encourage making better options more often and having cheat meals in tiny quantities and only on rare occasions. It cannot be argued that making better dietary choices is critical for controlling diabetes and lowering your risk of complications such as strokes and heart attacks, as well as other health conditions such as certain cancers.

Diet is essential for the overall control of diabetes, but a diagnosis of diabetes does not mean you have to be reduced to a life of bland and flavorless food. In fact, you should eat meals that are dense with nutrients and are based on a combination of complex carbohydrates, proteins, and healthy fats.

In this book, you will find some of the healthiest recipes for breakfast, lunch, dinner, dessert, snacks, soups and many more, so when it comes to eating, planning ahead may help you feel less anxious and more in control.

Chapter 1: Difference between Type 1 and Type 2 Diabetes

1.1 Diabetes

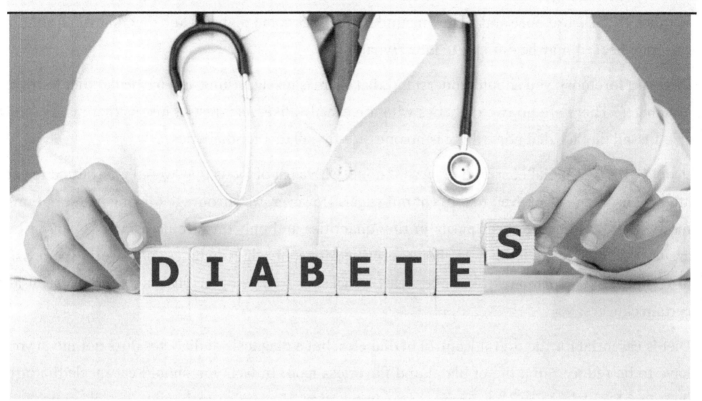

Diabetes is a long-term illness that affects the way your body converts food into energy. The majority of the food you consume is converted to sugar (also known as glucose) and absorbed into your circulation. When your blood sugar levels rise, your pancreas gets prompted to release insulin. Insulin is a key that allows blood sugar to enter your body's cells and be used as energy. If you are diagnosed with diabetes, your body either does not make enough insulin or does not utilize it the way it should. When there isn't enough insulin produced or when cells stop responding to insulin, then a large amount of blood sugar persists in your bloodstream. Over time, this can lead to major health issues like eyesight loss, heart disease, and renal illness. Although there is no treatment for diabetes at this time, decreasing weight, eating nutritious foods, and being active can all help.

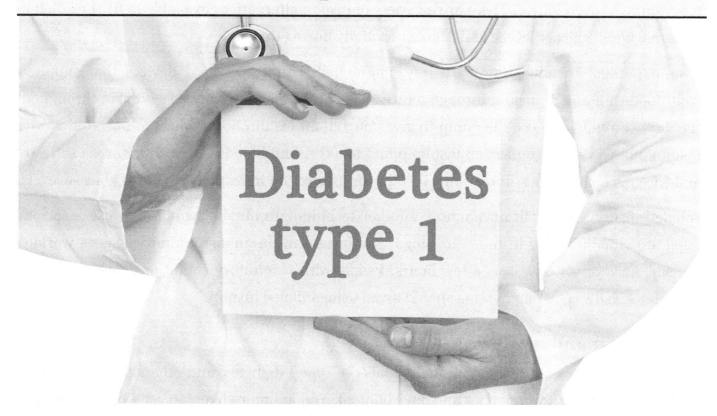

What is it?

In Type 1 diabetes, the immune system attacks the insulin-producing cells of the pancreas. The pancreas does not generate insulin as a result. Blood glucose levels rise without insulin, which is the key issue that doctors check for when diagnosing diabetes. Insulin injections are required for people with Type 1 diabetes to replace or mimic their natural insulin.

When it is usually diagnosed?

Type 1 diabetes affects the majority of individuals while they are kids and young adults.

What is the treatment for it?

People with Type 1 diabetes must take insulin from the start of their diagnosis. To put it another way, insulin therapy is required for survival. Anyone who uses insulin must monitor their blood glucose levels frequently to match the insulin they require with the insulin they are using.

Insulin injections: Most persons with Type 1 diabetes inject insulin into fatty tissues beneath their skin with a syringe, needle, or prefilled injection pen. Insulin is available in a variety of forms that last for varying amounts of time. Short-acting insulin kicks in after 15 minutes and lasts 2 to 4 hours. Other forms of insulin work over a longer period, such as six hours, twelve hours, twenty-four hours, or even longer. There are a variety of insulin alternatives available to fit your dietary patterns, blood glucose levels, and degree of activity during the day.

Insulin pumps: Insulin pumps are tiny, automated, battery-powered devices that supply a continuous amount of insulin through a little plastic tube that stays under your skin throughout the day. You may also use the pump to give yourself an insulin boost when you need it. Newer insulin pump systems connect an insulin pump to a constant blood glucose monitor via software and wireless technologies, automating insulin administration in response to blood glucose levels.

Inhaled insulin: Although uncommon, another technique to obtain insulin is to use a specific apparatus for breathing it into your lungs. The insulin in the inhalation device starts working quickly; however, it only lasts a few hours. People with respiratory conditions such as chronic bronchitis, asthma, or emphysema should avoid using inhaled insulin.

Who gets it and why?

Researchers are not sure why some individuals get Type 1 diabetes, and others do not. It's most likely the result of a mix of genes and environment. You are more likely to get Type 1 diabetes if you have a close relative who has it. Scientists are still investigating whether specific viruses contracted during pregnancy or early childhood might cause pancreatic damage, which leads to Type 1 diabetes.

Why does it matter?

Simply put, untreated diabetes can lead to death. Diabetic ketoacidosis (DKA) is a life-threatening condition that can occur if someone with Type 1 diabetes does not get enough insulin therapy for an extended time. Among the signs and symptoms are:

- Rapid heartbeat
- Shortness of breath
- Confusion
- Smell or fruity taste on the breath
- Coma

In the hospital, DKA must be handled as an emergency.

Higher blood glucose levels than normal might cause a variety of health concerns in the long run, even if they are not an emergency like DKA. High blood glucose levels damage blood arteries and nerves in the body. Diabetes patients commonly experience the following health issues:

- Blindness as a result of eye damage
- Renal failure occurs as a result of kidney injury.
- Neuropathy (nerve injury) causes numbness and discomfort in the hands and feet.
- Heart disease and mortality from heart disorders are at an increased (doubled) risk.
- Elevated risk of strokes (and stroke-related disability) and death

Keeping the blood glucose levels as close to normal as possible will help you avoid these problems.

How common is type 1 diabetes

Type 1 diabetes is less common than Type 2 diabetes. Type 1 diabetes affects just approximately 5% of persons with diabetes.

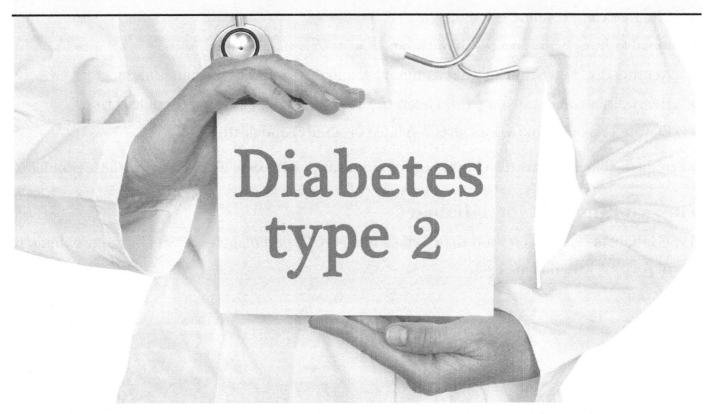

What is it?

Diabetes type 2 is the most frequent kind of diabetes. The pancreas generates insulin in Type 2 diabetes, but the body does not react to it normally. The primary distinction between T1D and T2D is this.

Insulin permits your body to utilize glucose from the bloodstream for energy under normal circumstances. However, with Type 2 diabetes, your body begins to disregard insulin, and glucose remains in your bloodstream rather than being utilized for energy. This is known as "insulin resistance," and it generates elevated blood glucose levels, similar to Type 1 diabetes.

The pancreas activates into overdrive in the initial stages of Type 2 diabetes, pumping out more and more insulin in an attempt to overcome insulin resistance. The pancreas becomes worn out over time and struggles to make insulin. That's why, like those with T1D, some patients with Type 2 diabetes have to inject insulin injections for a long period.

When it is usually diagnosed?

Type 2 diabetes is usually diagnosed in adulthood. Obese children and teenagers, on the other hand, have a risk of developing Type 2 diabetes at an early age.

What is the treatment for it?

Being physically active, eating healthy, and weight management are the keys to controlling Type 2 diabetes.

Healthy Nutrition: Eat a mix of fruits and vegetables, low-fat or fat-free dairy foods, whole grains, and lean meats for a healthy diet. Keep track of your portion sizes and avoid "empty" calories from sugary meals and beverages.

Physical activity: Since your muscles utilize glucose for fuel, being active during the day and doing regular exercise will reduce your blood glucose. Aim for 150 minutes of activity each week, which translates to 30 minutes five days a week.

Weight loss: Eating better and exercising more will help you lose extra pounds, which will assist in reducing blood glucose levels and halt the progression of Type 2 diabetes.

Many patients with Type 2 diabetes take medications to decrease their blood glucose levels in addition to adopting lifestyle modifications. The following are the most often prescribed drugs for Type 2 diabetes:

- Sulfonylureas (pill)
- Metformin (pill)
- Insulin (injections)
- DPP-4 inhibitors (pill)
- GLP-1 agonists (injections)
- SGLT2 inhibitors (pill)

Who gets it and why?

If you do any of the following risk factors, you're more likely to acquire Type 2 diabetes:

- If you're 45 years old or older, you're an older person.
- Obesity (BMI of 25 or above) is defined as being overweight or obese.
- Blood pressure that is too high
- Attempt to exercise no more than three times each week.
- A prediabetes diagnosis
- Type 2 diabetes in a parent or sibling

For women only:

- A polycystic ovary syndrome diagnosis (PCOS)
- Pregnancy and diabetes
- A baby weighing more than 9 pounds was born to her.

Why does it matter?

The hyperosmolar hyperglycemic state also known as HHS is a life-threatening syndrome that occurs when blood glucose levels are extremely high in people with Type 2 diabetes. In many aspects, it resembles DKA, the T1D medical emergency. Among the signs and symptoms are:

- Increased urination and thirst
- Dry mouth
- Weakness
- Confusion
- Rapid heartbeat
- Coma or death

An infection (such as pneumonia) or another sickness frequently causes HHS. HHS patients should be admitted to the hospital and treated as an emergency. Type 2 diabetes has the same long-term problems as Type 1 diabetes in terms of complications.

How common is it?

Type 2 diabetes affects around 90 percent to 95 percent of diabetics

Chapter 2: What Is Type 2 Diabetes?

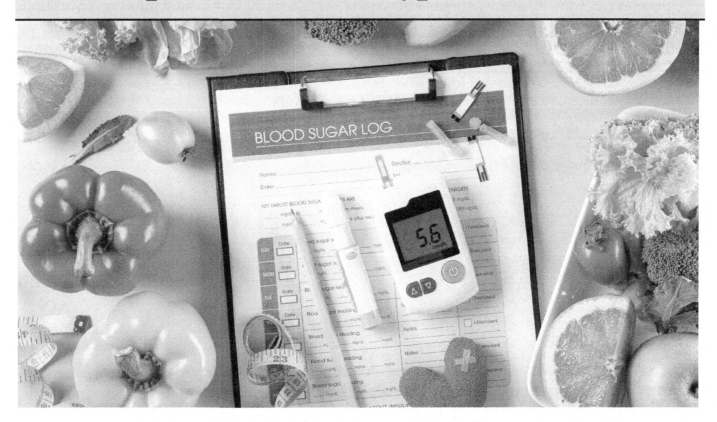

Type 2 diabetes is a disease in which the body grows resistant to the effects of insulin, and the pancreas' ability to generate enough insulin steadily declines. The illness is connected with non-modifiable genetic and family-related risk factors and modifiable lifestyle risk factors. The specific genetic origins of type 2 diabetes are unknown. Through dietary adjustments and increased physical activity, people may be able to greatly reduce or even stop the progression of the disease.

Type 2 Diabetes

- It is diagnosed whenever the pancreas does not create enough insulin (lower insulin production), the insulin does not operate well, or the body's cells do not respond well to insulin (also named insulin resistance)
- It accounts for 85–90% of all diabetes cases.
- Usually affects persons over 45 years of age, although it's becoming more common in younger age groups, including adolescents, children, and young adults.
- It is more common in those with a genetic history of diabetes or from certain ethnic groups.
- A complication of diabetes, such as visual issues, heart attack, or a foot ulcer, may be the first warning for some.

- It is treated with a mix of regular exercise, a nutritious diet, and weight loss. Because type 2 diabetes can worsen, many patients will require oral drugs and/or insulin injections over time, in addition to lifestyle adjustments.

Chapter 3: How to Control Type 2 Diabetes with Nutrition?

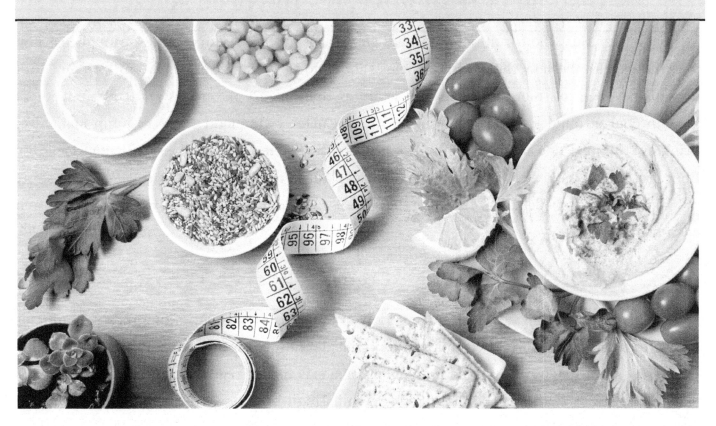

Healthy carbohydrates like vegetables, fruits, and whole grains; heart-healthy fish like mackerel, salmon, sardines, and tuna; low-fat dairy; and excellent fats like avocados, nuts, and olive oil are all part of a healthy type 2 diabetic diet. When diagnosed with diabetes, though, it's not just about eating the proper meals; it's also about restricting or avoiding items that might spike your blood sugar and put you at risk of problems.

"For overall balanced blood sugar regulation, it's all about moderation and making smart dietary choices," explains Amy Kimberlain.

"You should eat a well-balanced, healthy diet and stay away from processed carbs, which elevate blood sugar levels." You should also avoid saturated fat, which may be found in full-fat dairy, fatty meats, and fried meals because persons with type 2 diabetes are more likely to develop heart disease."

According to the American Diabetic Association, a balanced diabetes diet may help you control your weight or lose weight if you're overweight, which is significant because decreasing only 10 to 15 pounds can help you manage and prevent high blood sugar.

According to Kimberlain, decreasing weight can assist increase insulin sensitivity, which means you're less resistant to insulin and better equipped to respond to it.

Instead of fruit juice, try flavored seltzer

Although fiber-rich whole fruits are known as good carbs for those with diabetes, fruit juice is not. According to Kimberlain, those with diabetes should not drink juice, especially 100 percent fruit juice. Fruit juice has more minerals and vitamins than sugary beverages and soda, but juices contain concentrated levels of fruit sugar, which causes your blood sugar to jump fast. Also, drinking fruit juice doesn't fill you fully as much as eating a piece of fruit does since juice lacks the fiber present in whole fruit. Choose a zero-calorie plain or naturally flavored seltzer with a spray of lemon or lime for a delicious drink. Kimberlain also recommends infusing water with mint and cucumber.

Instead of dried fruit, eat fresh fruit

Although dried fruit provides fiber and a variety of minerals, the dehydration process eliminates the water, making it simpler to consume more - consider how many more raisins you can consume than grapes. Although eating dried apricots or raisins is healthier for you than eating a cookie, your blood sugar will still spike. Prefer whole fruits high in fiber instead of dried fruit, which induce a lower and slower spike in blood sugar.

Whole Grains Should Be Used Instead of White Carbs

Refined carbohydrates, such as white rice and anything produced with white flour, such as white bread and pasta, are major offenders on the low-quality carb list. Once your body begins to absorb these "white" carbohydrates, they function similarly to sugar, causing your glucose levels to rise. Whole grains, like wild or brown rice, oatmeal, barley, whole-grain bread, and high-fiber cereals, break down very slowly and have a less significant effect on blood sugar than white carbohydrates. "The first component should be a whole grain," Kimberlain adds. "Whether it's whole rye or whole grain, it should state 'whole."

Consume Low-fat dairy products instead of full-fat dairy products

You've undoubtedly heard that saturated fats found in dairy products can elevate your LDL cholesterol and put you at risk for heart disease. On the other hand, Saturated fats may still present another severe concern for diabetics: evidence suggests that eating a high-saturated-fat diet might increase insulin resistance. Full-fat dairy products manufactured with whole milk, such as cream, ice cream, full-fat yogurt, cream cheese, and other full-fat cheeses, should be avoided as much as possible. Instead, look for low-fat or fat-free dairy products. According to the American Heart Association, patients with type 2 diabetes should consume no more than 5 to 6 percent of the overall calories from saturated fat, and this advice is even more significant. So, if you eat 2,000 calories a day, saturated fat accounts for about 120 calories or 13 grams.

Choose lean proteins over fatty meat cuts

High-fat cuts of meat, like bologna, regular ground beef, sausage, hot dogs, ribs, and bacon should be limited or avoided by people with type 2 diabetes since, like full-fat dairy, they're high in saturated fats, adds Kimberlain. Saturated fats present in meat raise cholesterol and increase levels of inflammation in the body, and they can put make with diabetes at an even higher risk of heart disease than the general population because their risk is already high due to diabetes. Choose lean proteins such as skinless turkey and chicken, shellfish and fish, lean beef and pork tenderloin instead of fatty cuts of meat. When it comes to ground beef, Kimberlain recommends choosing meat that is at least 92 % lean and 8% fat.

Chapter 4: Foods to Avoid and Why?

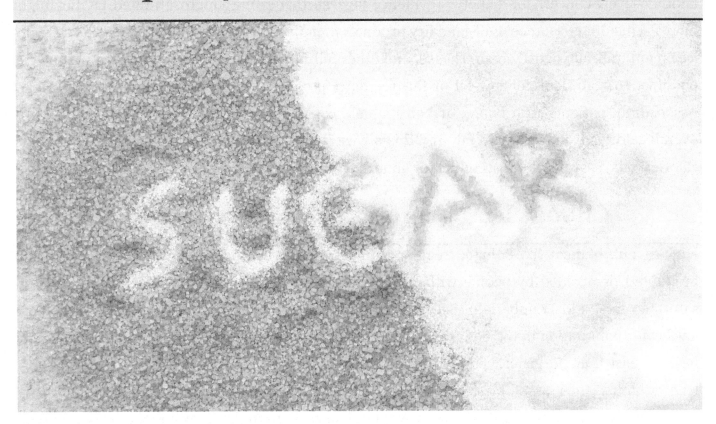

Diabetes is a chronic condition that has become a pandemic in adults and children worldwide. Diabetes that is not well controlled can lead to heart disease, blindness, renal disease, and other issues. Importantly, certain meals can elevate blood sugar and insulin levels, as well as induce inflammation, thereby increasing your disease risk. This topic contains a list of foods and beverages that people suffering from type 2 diabetes should avoid.

The macronutrients that supply energy to your body include carbohydrates, protein, and fat. Carbs, by far, have the largest impact on your blood sugar. This is because they are broken down into sugar and absorbed into circulation. Starches, sugar, and fiber are all examples of carbohydrates. Fiber, on the other hand, isn't digested and is instead absorbed by your body like other carbohydrates, so it doesn't boost your blood sugar. A meal's digestible or net carb content is calculated by subtracting fiber from the total carbohydrates in a serving. For example, a cup of mixed vegetables with 10 grams of carbohydrates and 4 grams of fiber has a net carb total of 6 grams. When people with diabetes eat too many carbohydrates at once, their blood sugar levels can be dangerously high. High amounts can harm your body's neurons and blood vessels over time, potentially leading to heart disease, renal illness, and other significant health problems. Low carbohydrate consumption can help avoid blood sugar increases and lower the risk of diabetic complications.

Below are the foods and drinks you should avoid consuming if you are suffering from type 2 diabetes.

4.1: Beverages with added sugar

Sugary beverages are by far the worst drinks for diabetics to consume.

For example, they're rich in carbohydrates, with 38.5 grams in a 12-ounce (354-mL) can of cola. Each serving of sweetened iced tea and lemonade has over 45 grams of carbohydrates derived only from sugar.

Furthermore, these beverages are high in fructose, which has been related to insulin resistance and diabetes. According to research, sugar-sweetened drinks have been linked to an increased risk of diabetes-related illnesses such as fatty liver disease.

In addition, sugary beverages' high fructose content may cause metabolic alterations that increase belly fat and possibly dangerous triglyceride and cholesterol levels.

In different research ingesting 25% of calories from high fructose drinks on a weight-maintenance diet resulted in increased insulin resistance and abdominal obesity, a reduced metabolic rate, and poorer heart health indicators in individuals with overweight and obesity

Instead of sugary beverages, drink water, unsweetened iced tea, or club soda to help manage blood sugar levels and reduce illness risk.

4.2: Trans Fats

Tran's fats that have been manufactured are exceedingly harmful. They're made by making unsaturated fatty acids more stable by adding hydrogen. Margarine, creamers, spreads, peanut butter, and frozen meals all include Tran's fats. Furthermore, they are frequently added to muffins, crackers, and other baked items to help increase the product's shelf life.

4.3: Pasta, White Bread, and Rice

Processed foods like rice, white bread, and pasta are rich in carbs. In persons with type 2 diabetes, eating bagels, bread, and other refined-flour items has been proven to drastically raise blood sugar levels. This reaction isn't limited to refined white flour-based items. Gluten-free pasta was also found to elevate blood sugar levels in one research, with rice-based varieties having the biggest effect.

In another study, high-carbohydrate diets elevated blood sugar levels and reduced brain function in persons with type 2 diabetes.

Fiber is scarce in these processed meals. Fiber aids in the slowing of sugar absorption into circulation. In other studies, substituting low-fiber diets with high-fiber foods was proven to lower blood sugar levels in diabetics considerably. Furthermore, patients with diabetes saw their cholesterol levels drop. Increased fiber consumption increased gut microbiota, which may have resulted in a reduction in insulin resistance.

4.4: Fruit-flavored yogurt

Plain Greek yogurt can be a healthy choice for diabetics. Fruit-flavored versions, on the other hand, are a different story.

Flavored yogurts are usually manufactured with nonfat or reduced fat milk and are high in carbohydrates and sugar.

In fact, a 1-cup serving of fruit-flavored yogurt might have roughly 31 grams of sugar, accounting for approximately 61 percent of the calories.

Frozen yogurt is widely regarded as a healthier alternative to ice cream. It can, however, contain just as much, if not more, sugar as ice cream. Rather than picking high-sugar yogurts that can cause blood sugar and insulin spikes, go for plain, whole milk yogurt, which has no added sugar and may help with appetite management, weight loss, and gastrointestinal health.

4.5: Sweetened breakfast cereals

If you have diabetes, cereal is one of the worst options to start your day.

Despite the health assurances on their labels, most cereals are heavily processed and contain significantly more carbohydrates than many consumers realize.

Furthermore, they contain very little protein, a nutrient that can make you feel satisfied and full throughout the day while keeping your blood sugar levels consistent.

Even certain "healthy" breakfast cereals are not recommended for diabetics.

For instance, granola has 44 grams of carbohydrates per 1/2-cup serving, whereas Grape Nuts have 47 grams. Furthermore, each serving contains no more than 7 grams of protein.

Skip most cereals in favor of a protein-based, low-carb breakfast to keep blood sugar and appetite under control.

4.6: Flavored coffee drinks

Coffee has been linked to a number of health advantages, including a lower diabetes risk.

Flavored coffee drinks, on the other hand, should be considered a liquid treat rather than a nutritious beverage. According to studies, your brain does not handle liquid and solid foods in the same way. When you drink calories, you don't make up for it later by eating less, which might contribute to weight gain.

Flavored coffee drinks have an abundance of carbohydrates in them. For example, a 16-ounce Caramel Frappuccino from Starbucks has 57 grams of carbohydrates, whereas a Blonde Vanilla Latte of the same size has 30 grams.

Choose regular coffee or espresso with a spoonful of half-and-half cream or heavy cream to keep your blood sugar in check and avoid weight gain.

4.7: French fries

French fries are a snack you should avoid if you have diabetes. Carbohydrate content in potatoes is rather high. A medium potato has 34.8 grams of carbohydrates with 2.4 grams of fiber.

Potatoes, on the other hand, may do more than raise your blood sugar once peeled and cooked in vegetable oil. Deep-frying meals have been demonstrated to create hazardous substances such as aldehydes and advanced glycation end products (AGEs) in excessive quantities. These substances may enhance the risk of illness by promoting inflammation.

Indeed, frequent consumption of French fries and other fried meals has been related to heart disease and cancer in various studies.

If you don't want to completely eliminate potatoes, a modest dish of sweet potatoes is the best alternative.

4.8: Processed meats

Sodium, preservatives, and other toxic substances are abundant in processed meats such as hot dogs, bacon, salami, and cold cuts. Additionally, processed meats have been linked to an increased risk of heart disease.

4.9: Fruit juice

Although fruit juice is frequently regarded as a healthful beverage, its blood sugar effects are comparable to those of sugary beverages and sodas.

This applies to both unsweetened 100 percent fruit juice and juice with added sugar. Fruit juice has a greater sugar and carb content than soda in some cases.

8 ounces of soda and 8 ounces of apple juice, for example, contain 22 and 24 grams of sugar, respectively. Grape juice has 35 grams of sugar in an equal serving.

Fruit juice, like sugar-sweetened drinks, is high in fructose. Obesity, Insulin Resistance, and heart disease are all caused by fructose.

Water with a slice of lemon is a far better option, as it contains less than 1 gram of carbohydrates and is almost calorie-free.

4.10: Packaged Snacks

Snacks such as crackers, pretzels, and other packaged meals are not recommended for individuals having type 2 diabetes.

They're usually produced with refined flour and contain few nutrients, but they're high in fast-digesting carbohydrates that spike blood sugar quickly.

The carbohydrate content of a 1-ounce (28-gram) portion of various popular snacks is as follows:

- Saltine crackers: 20.7 grams of carbohydrates in saltine crackers, containing 0.78 grams of fiber.
- Pretzels: 22.5 grams of carbohydrates in pretzels, including 0.95 grams of fiber.
- Graham crackers: 21.7 grams of carbohydrates, including 0.95 grams of fiber in graham crackers.

In fact, several of these meals may have even more carbohydrates than their nutrition labels indicate. According to one research, snack items include 7.7% more carbohydrates on average than the label claims.

If you're hungry in between meals, almonds or a few low-carb veggies with an ounce of cheese are a better option.

4.11: Dried fruits

Fruit is high in vitamin C and potassium, as well as other vital vitamins and minerals.

When Fruit is dried, it causes a loss of water, resulting in even larger quantities of essential nutrients. Unfortunately, the amount of sugar in it increases as well.

Grapes include 27.3 grams of carbohydrates per cup, with 1.4 grams of fiber. 1 cup of raisins, on the other hand, has 115 grams of carbohydrates, with 5.4 grams of fiber.

As a result, raisins have more than four times the amount of carbohydrates as grapes. The Carbohydrate content of other varieties of dried fruit is similar to that of fresh fruit.

You don't have to give up fruit entirely if you have diabetes. Sticking to low-sugar foods like small apples or fresh berries will help you maintain a healthy blood sugar level while staying within the goal range.

Chapter 5: How to Combine a Healthy Diet with Exercise?

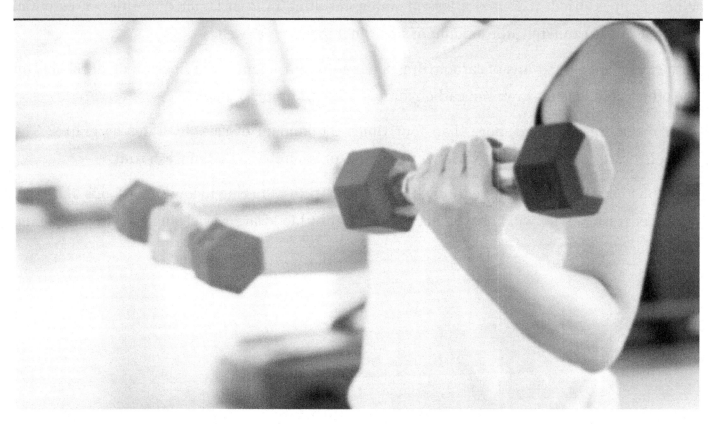

Diet and exercise are essential components of an effective diabetes prevention or management approach. Studies demonstrate that a healthy diet and regular exercise can significantly reduce the risk of diabetes, even in persons who are at high risk.

Other studies have found that lifestyle therapies such as exercise, nutrition, and education can assist people with type 2 diabetes reduce their blood sugar levels and improving risk factors linked with cardiovascular disease.

So, not only can eating a nutritious diet and doing adequate exercise help control blood sugar if you have type 2 diabetes, but it can also assist with weight reduction and high cholesterol—two concerns that are frequently associated with the diagnosis of type 2 diabetes.

A big clinical trial conducted by the National Institute of Diabetes followed people at risk for diabetes for three years and discovered that doing 150 minutes of exercise each week cut their risk of type 2 diabetes by 58 percent.

This indicates that maintaining a healthy lifestyle that includes physical activity, and nutritious food will help people avoid or reverse type 2 diabetes today and in the future.

5.1: Exercise: Start with the basics

While a doctor or dietitian may occasionally customize your diet to your needs (i.e., you can't handle gluten, you focus on low carb, you're a vegan, etc.), the sort of exercise that can help you avoid or manage type 2 diabetes is a little more varied.

Basically, any form of exercise is beneficial! Especially since doing something you like makes it easier to keep going. According to the American Heart Association, most individuals require at least 150 minutes of moderate aerobic physical exercise or 75 minutes of strenuous aerobic physical activity each week.

For example, two 30-minute powerwalks two days a week may be mixed with two 20-minute runs on the other days of the week. Keep in mind that moderate aerobic activity raises your heart rate, so make those powerwalks as brisk as possible!

Even low-volume activity increases insulin action in formerly sedentary people, according to the American Diabetes Association.

If you have type 2 diabetes, the benefits of exercise on blood sugar might be instantaneous. If you check your blood sugar prior, to and after 20 to 30 minutes of heart-pumping activity, you'll almost certainly detect a decrease.

Whether you're trying to avoid or manage a type 2 diabetes diagnosis, talk to your doctor before beginning a new fitness regimen, especially if exercise hasn't been a priority in your life until now. There may be health problems to consider based on where you are with your diagnosis.

5.2: Make exercise goals that are achievable

Inactivity is frequently linked to type 2 diabetes. If the prospect of exercising intimidates you or you struggle to keep to a regimen, here are a few tips to help you succeed:

- **Make an exercise schedule**

Schedule a workout for Sunday evening on your calendar. Create time blocks for your exercises like you do for washing, cooking, or work meetings.

- **Make an accountability system**

Having a support system will greatly help you remain on track on the days you don't feel inspired to work out, whether you find a companion to walk with in the park or hire a personal trainer at the gym.

- **Begin with a modest activity**

While the ultimate objective is to move your body for at least 30 minutes five days a week, the key is to start small. If you're currently working out for 20 minutes once a week, don't try to increase it to five days right once.

Increase the number of days and hours by one each week. For example, you may decide to exercise two days a week for 20 minutes in the first week, three days a week for 20 minutes in the third week, and four days a week for 20 minutes in the fourth week.

5.3: Which is better: Aerobic exercise or weight training?

While any activity that lasts at least 150 minutes per week is advantageous for persons who wish to avoid or control type 2 diabetes, combining two different forms of exercise may be the best option.

Aerobic exercise includes vigorous walking, jogging, swimming, dance, tennis, basketball, and other activities. Strength training, often known as resistance training, is a type of exercise that focuses on increasing or maintaining muscle mass and can be done with either body weight or weights.

These exercises are all beneficial in controlling blood sugar and cholesterol levels while also promoting weight reduction. However, research suggests that combining both may be the most effective workout strategy for type 2 diabetes glucose and lipid management.

Consider speaking with a physical therapist or a professional trainer about an exercise program that mixes aerobic activity and weight training. They can assist you in finding classes or creating a personalized plan to help you achieve your objectives.

5.4: Making a commitment to your exercise routine

Committing to a regular workout regimen may involve some time management and effort for some people. Others may want a little additional encouragement to keep motivated. Regardless of whatever group you fall into, the activities that offer you joy and make you feel encouraged are the ones for you.

If you need even more motivation, small research from 2008 found that after people with chronic tiredness completed working out, they felt less exhausted than others who had spent the same period sitting on the sofa. So, while exercise may appear to be chores at first, those who continue with it frequently discover that they begin to look forward to their activity.

It's not simple to change your way of life. It may be difficult at first, and you may need to restart. The good news is that type 2 diabetes is a chronic illness that may be prevented and even cured by making gradual lifestyle adjustments

Chapter 6: Breakfast Recipes

Breakfast is rightfully referred to be "the most essential meal of the day." Breakfast, as the name implies, is a meal that breaks the overnight fast. It replaces the glucose supply and helps you feel more alert and energetic. It also supplies other vital nutrients for better health.

Breakfast offers several health advantages. It boosts your energy and concentration in the near term, and it can help you lose weight and lessen your risk of type 2 diabetes and heart problems in the long run.

A meal that is full of fiber but low in added sugar, carbs, and salt is the ideal option. Nutrient-dense foods offer a sensation of fullness, which might make it easier for people to avoid unhealthful snacking.

In this chapter, you'll find several healthy and delicious breakfast choices for people with type-2 diabetes.

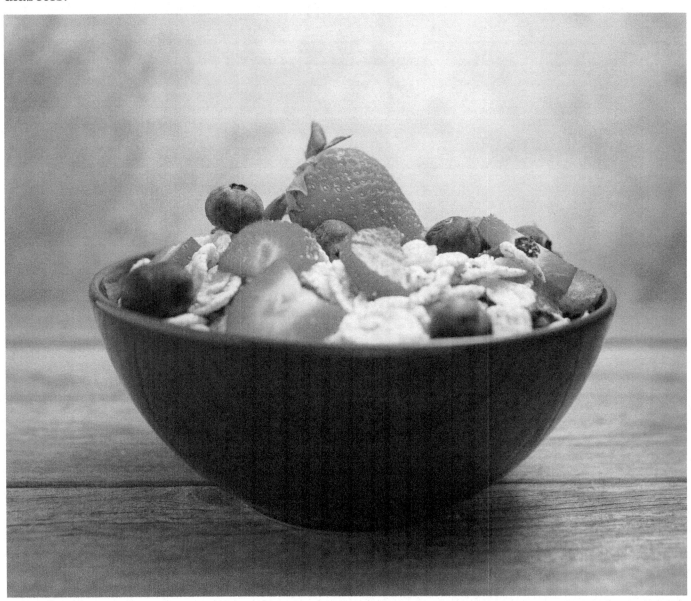

Mixed Berry Smoothie

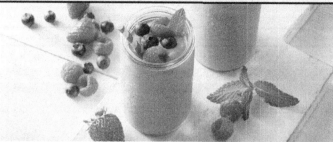

Total Time: 5 mins / **Prep. Time:** 5 mins /**Cooking Time:** N/A /**Difficulty:** Easy

Serving Size: 1 serving

Ingredients:

- 1 cup plain Greek yogurt
- 1 tbsp. sweetener
- 1 cup mixed berries, frozen
- 2 tbsp. nonfat milk

Instructions:

In a blender, combine all of the ingredients. Blend until completely smooth.

Nutritional Values: Calories: 205 kcal /Carbohydrates: 30 g /Protein: 22 g /Fat: 0 g/Sodium: 100 mg

Yogurt Pancakes

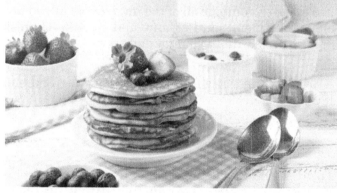

Total Time: 30 mins / **Prep. Time:** 25 mins /**Cooking Time:** 5 mins /**Difficulty:** Easy /**Serving Size:** 12 servings

Ingredients:

- 2 cups all-purpose flour
- ¼ cup water
- 2 tsp. baking powder
- 2 tbsp. sugar
- 2 large eggs, lightly beaten
- 1 tsp. baking soda
- 2 cups plain yogurt
- chocolate chips, sliced ripe bananas, dried cranberries, and chopped pecans (optional)

Instructions:

Combine the sugar, flour, baking soda, and baking powder in a small mixing dish. Whisk the yogurt, eggs, and water together in a separate dish. Stir in the dry ingredients till well combined and moistened.

Pour 1/4 cup of batter onto a heated griddle sprayed with cooking spray. Optional ingredients can be sprinkled on top if desired. Flip and cook till the other side is golden brown when bubbles appear on the surface.

Nutritional Values: Calories: 242 kcal /Carbohydrates: 40 g / Protein: 9 g /Fat: 5 g/Sodium: 432 mg

Quinoa Breakfast Bowl

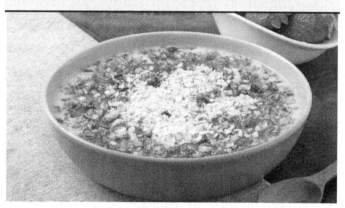

Total Time: 20 mins / **Prep. Time:** 5 mins /**Cooking Time:** 12-15 mins /**Difficulty:** Easy /**Serving Size:** 4 servings

Ingredients:

- 1 cup quinoa, rinsed
- 2 cups coconut milk
- Ground cinnamon, sugar substitute blend, vanilla Greek yogurt, brown sugar, honey, fresh blueberries, raisins, chia seeds, chopped apple (optional)

Instructions:

Bring milk to a boil in a large saucepan over medium heat, stirring regularly. Toss in the quinoa. Reduce heat to low and cook, covered, for 12-15 minutes, or until milk is absorbed. Remove the pan from the heat and fluff using a fork. Stir in your favorite combination of optional ingredients as desired.

Nutritional Values: Calories: 217 kcal

/Carbohydrates: 33 g /

Protein: 10 g /Fat: 5 g/Sodium: 59 mg

Whole Grain Banana Pancakes

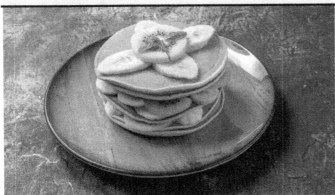

Total Time: 30 mins / **Prep. Time:** 25 mins /**Cooking Time:** 5 mins /**Difficulty:** Easy /**Serving Size:** 8 servings

Ingredients:

- 1 cup all-purpose flour
- 4 tsp. baking powder
- 2 cups milk, fat-free
- 1 cup whole wheat flour
- ½ tsp. salt
- 1 tsp. ground cinnamon
- 2 large eggs
- 1 tbsp. olive oil
- 2/3 cup mashed ripe banana
- 1 tbsp. maple syrup
- Additional syrup or sliced bananas (for garnish)
- ½ tsp. vanilla extract

Instructions:

Combine wheat flour, baking powder, salt, all-purpose flour, and ground cinnamon in a mixing bowl. Whisk together milk, eggs, oil, mashed banana, 1 tbsp. syrup, and vanilla in a separate bowl. Combine the wet and dry ingredients until moistened. Preheat a griddle that has been sprayed with nonstick cooking spray over medium flame. Cook about 1/4 cup of batter at a time until bubbles on the surface start to form, and the base is golden brown. Cook until pancakes are golden brown on the other side too. Serve with additional syrup and sliced bananas if desired.

Nutritional Values: Calories: 186 kcal /Carbohydrates: 32 g /Protein: 7 g /Fat: 4 g

Sodium: 392 mg

Chocolate Avocado Smoothie

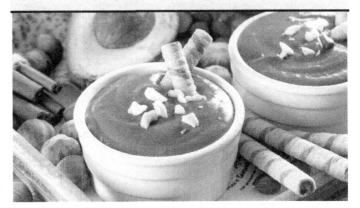

Total Time: 5 mins / **Prep. Time:** 5 mins /**Cooking Time:** N/A /**Difficulty:** Easy

Serving Size: 2 servings

Ingredients:

- ½ ripe avocado
- 1 cup coconut milk
- 3 tbsp. cocoa powder
- 1 tsp. lime juice
- ½ cup water
- 6-7 drops Stevia sweetener
- pinch of salt
- Fresh mint, for garnish

Instructions:

In a blender, combine all of the ingredients. Blend in a high-speed blend until creamy and smooth. Garnish the smoothie with fresh mint and serve.

Nutritional Values: Calories: 319 kcal /Carbohydrates: 12 g /Protein: 2 g /Fat: 30 g/Sodium: 180 mg

Hawaiian Hash

Total Time: 35 mins / **Prep. Time:** 20 mins /**Cooking Time:** 15 mins /**Difficulty:** Easy /**Serving Size:** 6 servings

Ingredients:

- 2 tsp. canola oil
- 4 cups sweet potatoes, cubed and peeled
- ½ cup sweet red pepper, chopped
- 1 cup onion, chopped
- 1 tsp. sesame oil
- ¼ cup water
- 1 tsp. fresh ginger root, minced

- 1 cup pineapple tidbits
- 1 cup cooked ham, cubed
- 1 tsp. soy sauce
- chopped fresh cilantro, for garnish
- ¼ cup salsa verde
- ½ tsp. black sesame seeds
- chopped macadamia nuts, for garnish

Instructions:

Heat the oils in a heavy skillet or big cast-iron pan over medium-high heat. Cook and stir for 5 minutes with the onion, sweet potatoes, pepper, and ginger root. Fill the pan halfway with water. Reduce heat to low and simmer for 8-10 minutes, or until potatoes are cooked, turning occasionally. Stir in the remaining ingredients, cook and stir for 2 minutes over medium-high heat or until well heated. Serve with cilantro and chopped macadamia nuts.

Nutritional Values: Calories: 158 kcal /Carbohydrates: 26 g /Protein: 7 g /Fat: 4 g /Sodium: 440 mg

Classic Avocado Toast

Total Time: 5 mins / **Prep. Time:** 5 mins /**Cooking Time:** N/A /**Difficulty:** Easy

Serving Size: 1 serving

Ingredients:

- 1 hearty bread slice, toasted
- ¼ medium ripe avocado, sliced
- 1/8 tsp. sea salt
- 2 tsp. olive oil

Instructions:

Spread olive oil over the bread and top with avocado slices. If desired, slightly mash the avocado and drizzle some more oil. Season the avocado toast with salt.

Nutritional Values: Calories: 160 kcal /Carbohydrates: 15 g /Protein: 3 g /Fat: 11 g

Sodium: 361 mg

Buttermilk Pumpkin Waffles

Total Time: 25 mins / **Prep. Time:** 20 mins /**Cooking Time:** 5 mins /**Difficulty:** Easy /**Serving Size:** 12 servings

Ingredients:

- ½ cup whole wheat flour
- 2 tbsp. brown sugar
- ¾ cup all-purpose flour
- 1 tsp. baking powder
- ½ tsp. ground ginger
- 1 tsp. ground cinnamon
- ¼ tsp. salt
- ¼ tsp. baking soda
- 2 large eggs, room temperature
- ¼ tsp. ground cloves
- 1¼ cups buttermilk
- 2 tbsp. butter, melted
- ½ cup fresh pumpkin
- maple syrup and butter (optional)

Instructions:

Combine the dry ingredients in a large mixing bowl. Whisk together the buttermilk, eggs, pumpkin, and melted butter in a small mixing dish. Just until the dry ingredients are moistened, stir in the wet components. Bake until golden brown in a preheated waffle machine according to the manufacturer's instructions. Serve with maple syrup and butter, if preferred.

Nutritional Values: Calories: 194 kcal /Carbohydrates: 28 g /Protein: 7 g /Fat: 6 g

Sodium: 325 mg

Southwest Breakfast Wraps

Total Time: 30 mins / **Prep. Time:** 20 mins /**Cooking Time:** 10 mins /**Difficulty:** Medium/**Serving Size:** 4 servings

Ingredients:

- 1 tbsp. olive oil
- ½ cup fresh mushrooms, sliced
- 1 medium red onion, chopped
- 1 sweet red pepper, chopped
- 1 small green pepper, chopped
- 4 oz. green chilies, chopped
- 4 whole wheat tortillas, toasted
- 1 jalapeno pepper, chopped
- 8 large egg whites
- 1 garlic clove, minced
- ¼ cup cheese blend, shredded

Instructions:

Heat the oil in a large nonstick skillet over medium-high heat. Cook and stir in the mushrooms, onion, chilies, peppers, and garlic until the peppers are crisp-tender. Remove from the pan and set aside. Beat egg whites and cheese together in a small bowl until well combined. Cook and whisk the egg white mixture in the pan over medium heat until the egg whites begin to solidify and there is no liquid egg left. Place a spoonful of the egg white mixture in the center of each tortilla, then top with the veggie mixture. Fold the tortilla's bottom and edges over the filling and roll it up.

Nutritional Values: Calories: 254 kcal /Carbohydrates: 29 g /Protein: 14 g /Fat: 8 g

Sodium: 446 mg

Smoothie Bowl with Berries

Total Time: 5 mins / **Prep. Time:** 5 mins /**Cooking Time:** N/A /**Difficulty:** Easy

Serving Size: 2 servings

Ingredients:

- ½ cup almond milk, unsweetened
- 3 cups crushed ice
- ¼ cup chopped strawberries
- ½ tsp. husk powder
- 1 tbsp. coconut oil
- 1/3 cup vanilla protein powder
- 5 drops Stevia sweetener
- Mixed berries, for garnish

Instructions:

In a blender, add the ice cubes and let them settle for 5 minutes. You want them to melt somewhat to provide traction for the blender. In a blender, combine the other ingredients and mix until creamy, smooth, and light pink. Transfer to a serving dish and top with mixed berries as garnish.

Nutritional Values: Calories: 166 kcal /Carbohydrates: 4 g /Protein: 17 g /Fat: 9 g

Sodium: 49 mg

Honey French Toast

Total Time: 25 mins / **Prep. Time:** 15 mins /**Cooking Time:** 10 mins /**Difficulty:** Easy /**Serving Size:** 6 servings

Ingredients:

- 1 cup low-fat milk
- 4 large eggs

- 1 tbsp. honey
- 1/8 tsp. pepper
- ½ tsp. ground cinnamon
- 12 slices whole wheat bread
- vanilla frosting or Cinnamon sugar (optional)

Instructions:

Whisk together the eggs, honey, milk, pepper, and cinnamon in a small bowl. Both sides of the bread should be dipped in the egg mixture. Cook 3-4 minutes per side on a greased hot griddle, or until golden brown. Top with vanilla icing or sprinkle with cinnamon sugar, if preferred.

Nutritional Values: Calories: 218 kcal /Carbohydrates: 28 g /Protein: 13 g /Fat: 6 g

Sodium: 331 mg

Vegetarian Lentils with Egg Toast

Total Time: 15 mins / **Prep. Time:** 5 mins /**Cooking Time:** 10 mins /**Difficulty:** Easy /**Serving Size:** 2 servings

Ingredients:

- 2 oz. vegetable broth, low-sodium
- 2 cloves garlic, minced
- 1 medium onion, diced
- ½ red bell pepper, sliced
- ¼ avocado, sliced
- ½ orange bell pepper, sliced
- ½ tsp. smoked paprika
- ½ yellow bell pepper, sliced
- 15 oz. sodium canned lentils, drained
- ½ tsp. garlic powder
- ground black pepper to taste
- ⅛ tsp. chipotle powder
- olive-oil spray
- 2 slices whole-grain bread
- 2 large eggs
- 2 tbsp. fresh parsley
- ½ lemon, sliced

Instructions:

Cook garlic and onions in vegetable stock over medium to high heat until transparent. Cook for another 3-4 minutes after adding the bell peppers. In a large mixing bowl, combine the lentils, chipotle powder, paprika, black pepper, and garlic powder. Reduce to medium-low heat and simmer for another 3-4 minutes, stirring periodically. Meanwhile, cut a hole in each piece of bread with a plain-edge tiny circular cutter; toast the bread. Spray a medium frying pan with cooking spray and fry eggs sunny-side up. Divide the lentil mixture onto two dishes and top with an egg and a toast with the hole cut out over the yolk on each. Garnish with lemon, avocado, and parsley on top of each plate. Lemon juice should be squeezed over the lentil mixture.

Nutritional Values: Calories: 420 kcal /Carbohydrates: 62 g /Protein: 25 g /Fat: 10 g

Sodium: 480 mg

Watermelon Smoothie

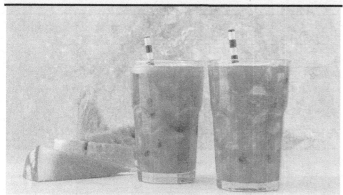

Total Time: 5 mins / **Prep. Time:** 5 mins /**Cooking Time:** N/A /**Difficulty:** Easy

Serving Size: 4 servings

Ingredients:

- 2 cups chilled watermelon, cubed
- 5 drops stevia sweetener
- 1 lime juice
- 10 fresh mint leaves
- ½ cup soy milk
- 3 cups ice

Instructions:

In a blender, combine the lime juice, watermelon, soy milk, stevia, and mint. Blend on high speed until absolutely smooth. Include the ice in the blender. Pulse briefly to incorporate the smoothie and serve immediately.

Nutritional Values: Calories: 33 kcal /Carbohydrates: 6 g /Protein: 1 g /Fat: 0.5 g

Sodium: 13 mg

Cinnamon Chia Seed Pudding

Total Time: 5 mins / **Prep. Time:** 5 mins /**Cooking Time:** N/A /**Difficulty:** Easy

Serving Size: 1 serving

Ingredients:

- 3 tbsp. chia seeds
- 1 tsp. maple syrup
- ¼ tsp. ground cinnamon
- ¾ cup almond milk, unsweetened
- 1 tbsp. slivered almonds

Instructions:

Combine almond milk and chia seeds in a small glass jar or container. Close the jar and shake it vigorously. Allow for a 5-minute rest period. Add ground cinnamon and maple syrup to the jar. Close the jar and shake it firmly to ensure that the seeds do not stick to the bottom. Place in the refrigerator for four hours or overnight. Take it out of the fridge. Slivered almonds should be sprinkled on top. Enjoy.

Nutritional Values: Calories: 293 kcal /Carbohydrates: 23 g /Protein: 12 g /Fat: 17.5 g/Sodium: 123 mg

Pumpkin Spice Smoothie

Total Time: 5 mins / **Prep. Time:** 5 mins /**Cooking Time:** N/A /**Difficulty:** Easy

Serving Size: 1 serving

Ingredients:

- 4 ice cubes
- 2 tbsp. almond butter
- ½ cup almond milk, unsweetened
- Pinch pumpkin pie spice
- 1 scoop Collagen Powder

Instructions:

In a blender jug, combine all ingredients and blend for 20-30 seconds. Serve immediately.

Nutritional Values: Calories: 355 kcal /Carbohydrates: 8 g /Protein: 18 g /Fat: 26 g

Sodium: 235 mg

Apple Pie Oats

Total Time: 10 mins / **Prep. Time:** 2 mins /**Cooking Time:** 8 mins /**Difficulty:** Easy

Serving Size: 4 servings

Ingredients:

- ¼ cup soy milk, unsweetened
- ⅓ cup whole grain oats
- ½ cup water
- 1 tbsp. chia seeds
- 8 walnuts, halved
- stevia to taste
- 1 small yellow opal apple
- Cinnamon pinch

Instructions:

Add milk, water, and oats to a small saucepan over medium heat. Mix until everything is well combined. For the next 3 minutes, stir constantly. Add the apple that has been cut. Mix until everything is well combined. Cook for another 2 minutes, and then turn off the heat. Chia seeds should be added to the oat mixture. Cook for another minute. Remove the pan from the heat. Serve with cinnamon, walnuts and stevia sprinkled on top.

Nutritional Values: Calories: 343 kcal /Carbohydrates: 41.5 g /Protein: 10 g /Fat: 16 g/Sodium: 29 mg

Butternut Squash Muffins

Total Time: 30 mins / **Prep. Time:** 10 mins /**Cooking Time:** 20 mins /**Difficulty:** Medium/**Serving Size:** 12 servings

Ingredients:

- ¾ cup butternut squash puree
- ½ cup vegetable oil
- ½ cup cinnamon apple sauce
- 2 eggs
- ¾ cup Truvia Cane Sugar Blend
- 1½ cups whole wheat flour
- ¾ tsp. salt
- 1 tsp. pumpkin spice
- 1 tsp. baking soda
- 2 tsp. ground cinnamon

Instructions:

Using nonstick cooking spray, coat the muffin pan. Combine the wet ingredients in a large mixing bowl: butternut squash puree, vegetable oil, eggs, and applesauce. Dry ingredients should be stirred together in a separate bowl. Combine the dry and wet ingredients in a mixing bowl and whisk until smooth. Fill every muffin cup 2/3 full with batter using a cookie scoop. Preheat the oven to 375°F and bake for 18–20 minutes. Enjoy.

Nutritional Values: Calories: 196 kcal /Carbohydrates: 27 g /Protein: 3 g /Fat: 10 g

Sodium: 297 mg

Cinnamon Breakfast Smoothie

Total Time: 5 mins / **Prep. Time:** 5 mins /**Cooking Time:** N/A /**Difficulty:** Easy

Serving Size: 1 serving

Ingredients:

- ½ cup coconut milk
- ½ tsp. cinnamon
- ¼ cup oats
- 1/3 cup vanilla Greek yogurt
- ¼ tsp. vanilla extract
- ½ frozen banana

Instructions:

In a blender, combine all of the ingredients and mix until smooth. Pour into a glass and enjoy.

Nutritional Values: Calories: 195 kcal /Carbohydrates: 34 g /Protein: 9 g /Fat: 3 g

Sodium: 48 mg

Low-Carb Green Smoothie

Total Time: 5 mins / **Prep. Time:** 5 mins /**Cooking Time:** N/A /**Difficulty:** Easy

Serving Size: 2 servings

Ingredients:

- 1 tbsp. almond butter
- Few drops Stevia sweetener
- ¼ cup protein powder
- 1 cup almond milk, unsweetened
- 1 tsp. vanilla extract
- ½ cup frozen avocado
- 2 cups spinach
- 1 cup ice cubes

Instructions:

All items except the ice cubes should be added to the blender. Blend until smooth. Blend in the ice cubes until fully smooth and creamy.

Nutritional Values: Calories: 185 kcal /Carbohydrates: 6 g /Protein: 16 g /Fat: 11 g

Sodium: 238 mg

Cauliflower Cups

Total Time: 40 mins / **Prep. Time:** 10 mins /**Cooking Time:** 30 mins /**Difficulty:** Medium/**Serving Size:** 12 servings

Ingredients:

- 3 cups riced cauliflower
- ¾ cup mozzarella cheese
- 3 eggs
- ¼ cup milk
- 2 tbsp. parmesan cheese
- 1/8 tsp. salt

Instructions:

Using nonstick cooking spray, coat the muffin pan. Combine all ingredients (except parmesan cheese) in a big mixing bowl. Fill every muffin cup 2/3 full with batter using a cookie scoop. Parmesan cheese should be sprinkled on top of each cauliflower cup. Preheat the oven to 350°F and bake for 30 minutes. While the cauliflower cups are still warm, enjoy them.

Nutritional Values: Calories: 51 kcal /Carbohydrates: 2 g /Protein: 10 g /Fat: 3 g

Sodium: 115 mg

Open Face Loaded Toast

Total Time: 25 mins / **Prep. Time:** 10 mins /**Cooking Time:** 15 mins /**Difficulty:** Easy /**Serving Size:** 1 serving

Ingredients:

- 1 slice bread, toasted
- ¼ avocado
- 1 hardboiled egg, sliced
- ¼ cup baby spinach
- 1 tbsp. capers
- Salt dash
- 3 cherry tomatoes
- ¼ cucumber, sliced
- dash of pepper

Instructions:

In a small saucepan, bring water to a boil. Cook an egg in boiling water for 12 minutes. When boiled, transfer it to an ice bath. Toast the bread in the meantime. On top, mash the avocado. Toss in the veggies and capers. On top, place a sliced egg. Season the toast with salt and pepper to taste.

Nutritional Values: Calories: 369 kcal /Carbohydrates: 30 g /Protein: 13 g /Fat: 27 g

Sodium: 1038 mg

Spanish Omelette

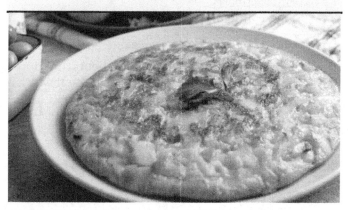

Total Time: 20 mins / **Prep. Time:** 5 mins /**Cooking Time:** 15 mins /**Difficulty:** Easy /**Serving Size:** 4 servings

Ingredients:

- 1 tbsp. vegetable oil
- 1 red pepper, chopped
- 2 medium onions, chopped
- 2 large potatoes, chopped and boiled
- 4 medium eggs
- 1 tbsp. chopped parsley
- Salt and black pepper, to taste

Instructions:

In a frying pan, heat 1 tbsp. of oil. Add onions and cook until the onions are tender. Cook for further 5 minutes after adding the red pepper. In a mixing dish, whisk together the eggs and season them with salt and pepper. Add the parsley, potatoes, and fried vegetables into the egg mixture. Pour the egg mixture onto the hot frying pan and evenly distribute it to the edges. Cook for 5 minutes, or until the egg mixture begins to pull away from the pan's edge. To cook the surface of the omelet, place the pan on a moderately preheated grill for about 3 minutes.

Nutritional Values: Calories: 172 kcal /Carbohydrates: 14 g /Protein: 8 g /Fat: 9 g

Sodium: 100 mg

Raspberry Smoothie

Total Time: 5 mins / **Prep. Time:** 5 mins
/**Cooking Time:** N/A /**Difficulty:** Easy

Serving Size: 2 Servings

Ingredients:

- 1½ cup coconut milk, unsweetened
- 1 medium avocado¾ cup raspberry
- 1 tbsp. lemon juice
- ¾ cup raspberry
- 1 scoop vanilla protein powder, sugar-free

Instructions:

In a blender, combine all of the ingredients and puree for around 30 seconds. Taste and adjust the flavor as needed, then serve right away.

Nutritional Values: Calories: 231 kcal /Carbohydrates: 13 g /Protein: 14 g /Fat: 14 g

Sodium: 32 mg

Raspberry Chia Pudding

Total Time: 4 hours 10 mins / **Prep. Time:** 10 mins /**Resting Time:** 4 hours **Cooking Time:** N/A mins /**Difficulty:** Easy /**Serving Size:** 2 servings

Ingredients:

- 4 tbsp. chia seeds
- 1 tbsp. maple syrup
- 1½ cups coconut milk
- 1 pinch salt
- 2 tbsp. walnuts
- 1 tsp. pure vanilla extract
- 2 + ½ cup fresh raspberries

Instructions:

Combine the coconut milk and chia seeds in a medium mixing bowl and toss thoroughly to avoid any lumps. Mix in the maple syrup, salt and vanilla extract very well. Cover the bowl with plastic wrap and place in the refrigerator for 4-5 hours. Alternatively, chill overnight. Puree 2 cups of raspberries in a blender after 4-5 hours. Place a layer of chia pudding in dessert glasses, followed by a layer of pureed raspberries. Serve the chia pudding with walnuts and raspberries on top.

Nutritional Values: Calories: 232 kcal /Carbohydrates: 30 g /Protein: 6 g /Fat: 10 g

Sodium: 36 mg

Brussels Sprouts Casserole

Total Time: 29 mins / **Prep. Time:** 10 mins
/**Cooking Time:** 19 mins /**Difficulty:** Medium
/**Serving Size:** 6 servings

Ingredients:

- 2 lb. Brussels sprouts
- ½ cup heavy cream
- 8 oz. cream cheese, softened
- ½ tsp. onion powder
- ½ tsp. garlic powder
- black pepper to taste
- Fresh parsley, chopped
- Salt to taste
- 1 cup mozzarella, shredded

Instructions:

Preheat the oven to 425°F with the oven rack in the middle position. Fill a big saucepan halfway with water and a steamer basket in the base to steam Brussels sprouts. Bring the water to a boiling point in a large pot. Fill the steamer basket halfway with Brussel sprouts. Cover and steam till the Brussels sprouts are fork tender, about 15 minutes. Meanwhile, combine heavy cream, cream cheese, onion powder, garlic powder, salt, and freshly ground black pepper in a large mixing bowl. To incorporate all of the ingredients, whisk them together thoroughly. Remove the Brussels sprouts from the steamer basket and toss them in a mixing dish with the cream cheese mixture. Allowing Brussels sprouts to cool isn't essential. Add the Brussels sprout mixture to an oiled casserole dish and top the Brussels sprout mixture with mozzarella cheese. Bake for 10 minutes, or until the cheese is melted and uncovered. Set the broiler on high for the last 3 minutes and broil the casserole. Keep a watchful eye on it to avoid it burning. Serve with fresh chopped parsley on top.

Nutritional Values: Calories: 286 kcal /Carbohydrates: 15 g /Protein: 12 g /Fat: 19 g

Sodium: 471 mg

Breakfast Egg Muffins

Total Time: 35 mins / **Prep. Time:** 10 mins
/**Cooking Time:** 25 mins /**Difficulty:**
Medium/**Serving Size:** 12 servings

Ingredients:

- 1 ½ cups cauliflower, finely chopped
- ¼ cup cooked ham, chopped
- 5 large eggs, beaten
- ½ cup red bell pepper, chopped
- ½ cup spinach, chopped
- ½ tsp. garlic powder
- ½ cup red onion, chopped
- kosher salt, to taste
- 1 cup Mozzarella cheese, shredded
- ½ tsp. dried oregano
- black pepper to taste

Instructions:

Preheat your oven to 375°F with a rack in the middle. Use a cooking spray to grease a muffin tray or brush muffin cups using olive oil or melted butter. Whisk the eggs vigorously in a large mixing dish. Cauliflower, spinach, ham, bell pepper, mozzarella, garlic powder, onion, dried oregano, salt, and black pepper should be combined in the same bowl. To combine, whisk everything together thoroughly. Fill every muffin cup three-quarters with batter. If desired, top with diced ham and more shredded cheese. Bake for 20-25 minutes till golden brown. Allow cooling for 5 minutes before loosening with a butter knife along the sides of each muffin. You may skip this step if you're using a silicone muffin pan/cup. Take them out of the pan and eat them.

Nutritional Values: Calories: 94 kcal /Carbohydrates: 2 g /Protein: 7 g /Fat: 6 g

Sodium: 426 mg

Avocado Smoothie

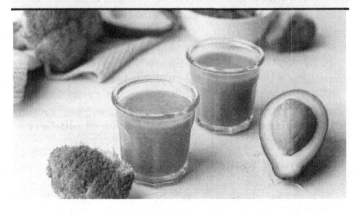

Total Time: 10 mins / **Prep. Time:** 10 mins /**Cooking Time:** N/A /**Difficulty:** Easy

Serving Size: 2 servings

Ingredients:

- 2 cups baby spinach

- 2 mint sprigs
- 1 cup baby kale
- 1 tbsp. fresh lemon juice
- 2 cups water
- 1 avocado, cubed
- ½ cup ice cubes

Instructions:

In a high-powered blender, add the kale, spinach, mint, lemon juice, avocado and water. Finally, add the ice cubes. Using a high-speed blender, blend the ingredients until smooth. Add a few drops of Stevia to sweeten the smoothie. Serve and enjoy.

Nutritional Values: Calories: 186 kcal /Carbohydrates: 12 g /Protein: 4 g /Fat: 14 g

Sodium: 70 mg

Vegetable Frittata

Total Time: 30 mins / **Prep. Time:** 10 mins /**Cooking Time:** 20 mins /**Difficulty:** Medium/**Serving Size:** 6 servings

Ingredients:

- 2 tbsp. olive oil
- ¼ cup fresh parsley, chopped
- 1 cup red onion, chopped
- ½ cup asparagus, chopped
- 1 cup frozen kale, chopped
- ½ cup almond milk
- 5 large eggs, lightly beaten
- ½ tsp. garlic powder
- 1 tsp. Italian seasoning
- 1 cup cherry tomatoes, halved
- ½ tsp. salt and black pepper
- ½ cup mozzarella cheese, shredded

Instructions:

Preheat the oven to 425°F. In a 10-inch cast iron skillet, heat the oil over medium-low heat. Combine the parsley, onion, asparagus, and kale in the pan. Cook occasionally stirring, for 3-5 minutes or until the vegetables are softened. Whisk together the almond milk, garlic powder, eggs, Italian seasoning, salt, and black pepper in a medium mixing bowl. Pour the prepared egg mixture into the sautéed vegetables, covering the vegetable mixture completely. Layer tomatoes on top of the egg mixture and top it with shredded mozzarella cheese. Bake the frittata for 15 minutes or until the frittata is fully cooked. The center should be firm, not swaying. Serve hot with a tasty salad. Enjoy.

Nutritional Values: Calories: 133 kcal /Carbohydrates: 4 g /Protein: 7 g /Fat: 10 g

Sodium: 124 mg

Blueberry Smoothie

Total Time: 5 mins / **Prep. Time:** 5 mins /**Cooking Time:** N/A /**Difficulty:** Easy

Serving Size: 2 servings

Ingredients:

- 1½ cup coconut milk, unsweetened
- ½ tsp. vanilla extract
- ½ cup blueberries
- ½ cup almond milk, unsweetened
- 4 tbsp. pea protein powder

Instructions:

In a high-speed blender, combine the almond milk, blueberries, vanilla, and pea protein powder. Add the coconut milk in smaller amounts until the smoothie reaches the desired consistency. Blend on high speed until all ingredients are well combined, and the smoothie has acquired a light purple color.

Nutritional Values: Calories: 402 kcal /Carbohydrates: 9 g /Protein: 14 g /Fat: 33 g

Sodium: 264 mg

Cranberry Orange Scones

Total Time: 40 mins / **Prep. Time:** 10 mins /**Cooking Time:** 20 mins /**Resting Time:** 10 mins **Difficulty:** Medium/**Serving Size:** 8 servings

Ingredients:

- 2 cups almond flour
- ½ tsp. baking powder
- 1/3 cup erythritol
- ¼ cup coconut oil, melted
- ¼ tsp. sea salt
- ½ tsp. vanilla extract
- 2 tbsp. orange zest
- ½ cup cranberries
- 1 large egg

Instructions:

Preheat the oven to 350°F. Use parchment paper to line a baking sheet. Combine the erythritol, almond flour, sea salt, and baking powder in a medium

mixing bowl. Whisk together the egg, vanilla, orange zest, and melted coconut oil in a small bowl. Using a spoon or spatula, press the wet mixture into the almond flour dry mixture until smooth dough forms. Stir in the cranberries and press them into the dough. Form a disc out of the dough in the prepared pan. Cut into 8 wedges as if you were making a pie or pizza. Separate the pieces by about 1 inch. Bake the scones for 18–22 minutes, or until golden brown. Allow cooling entirely on the pan so they become firm.

Nutritional Values: Calories: 232 kcal /Carbohydrates: 9 g /Protein: 6 g /Fat: 21 g

Sodium: 200 mg

Almond Flour Pancakes

Total Time: 30 mins / **Prep. Time:** 5 mins /**Cooking Time:** 25 mins /**Difficulty:** Medium/**Serving Size:** 5 servings

Ingredients:

- 2 large eggs
- 4 tbsp. peanut butter
- 2 tbsp. almond milk
- 1 tsp. baking powder
- 2/3 cup almond flour
- 2 tbsp. Natural Sweetener
- 2 tsp. vanilla extract
- Cooking spray

Instructions:

In a blender, combine all of the ingredients. For around 15 seconds, blend it. Stop a few times if necessary to scrape the corners of the blender bowl and ensure that all of the ingredients are properly blended. Spray a nonstick pan with cooking spray and heat to medium-low. Scoop the batter into the pan with a 1/4 measuring cup. Allow 2 to 3 minutes on each side to cook until the edges are crisp. Cook for an additional minute or two on the opposite side. Enjoy with your favorite toppings, such as blueberries with sugar-free syrup will work well.

Nutritional Values: Calories: 222 kcal /Carbohydrates: 11 g /Protein: 11 g /Fat: 15 g

Sodium: 105 mg

Cranberry Muffins

Total Time: 35 mins / **Prep. Time:** 10 mins /**Cooking Time:** 25 mins /**Difficulty:** Medium /**Serving Size:** 12 servings

Ingredients:

- 1 cup cranberries
- ½ cup + 1 tbsp. sweetener
- 1 tbsp. fresh lemon juice
- 3 eggs
- ½ cup applesauce, unsweetened
- 3 cups almond flour
- 1½ tsp. baking powder
- 1 tsp. vanilla extract
- ¼ tsp. salt
- ½ tsp. baking soda
- Dark chocolate, for drizzling

Instructions:

Preheat the oven to 350°F. Line a muffin tray using paper liners. Combine the lemon juice, cranberries, and 1 tbsp. of sweetener in a small bowl to prepare cranberry mixture. Applesauce, eggs, 1/2 cup sweetener, and vanilla extract should all be combined in a large mixing bowl. Mix everything together until it's completely smooth. Now add the baking powder, almond flour, salt and baking soda to a mixing bowl to prepare the batter. Combine the cranberry mixture in the prepared batter and fold it in. Divide the batter among the muffin cups that have been prepared. It's important to fill each muffin cup three-quarters full. Bake for 25-30 minutes, or until the muffins are golden brown on top and a wooden skewer inserted in the center comes out clean. Drizzle melted chocolate over the muffins after that. Enjoy.

Nutritional Values: Calories: 176 kcal /Carbohydrates: 8 g /Protein: 6 g /Fat: 14 g

Sodium: 127 mg

Flourless Banana Pancakes

Total Time: 30 mins / **Prep. Time:** 10 mins /**Cooking Time:** 20 mins /**Difficulty:** Medium/**Serving Size:** 4 servings

Ingredients:

- 2 medium bananas
- ¼ tsp. salt
- 1 tsp. vanilla extract
- 3 large eggs
- ½ tsp. baking powder
- ½ cup rolled oats
- ½ tsp. cinnamon

Instructions:

Mash the bananas using a fork in a large mixing dish until nearly smooth. Some lumps are normal. Whisk together the vanilla extract with eggs. Combine the baking powder, oats, salt, and cinnamon in a mixing bowl. Stir until everything is well incorporated. Heat a greased pan over medium heat while the pancake batter rests. 1/4 cup batter should be poured into the pan for each pancake. Cook the pancake for 3-4 minutes, or till bubbles begin to appear on the surface. Cook for a further 3-4 minutes after flipping the pancake. Remove the pan from the heat and set it aside. Continue with the remaining batter till you have a total of 8 pancakes.

Nutritional Values: Calories: 128 kcal /Carbohydrates: 17 g /Protein: 6 g /Fat: 4 g

Sodium: 260 mg

Cauliflower Fritters

Total Time: 40 mins / **Prep. Time:** 15 mins /**Cooking Time:** 25 mins /**Difficulty:** Medium /**Serving Size:** 12 servings

Ingredients:

- 1 large cauliflower
- ¼ cup almond flour
- 3 large eggs
- ½ cup white cheddar cheese, grated
- 1 tsp. garlic powder
- 2 tbsp. parmesan cheese, grated
- ½ tsp. pepper
- ½ tsp. salt
- 1 tbsp. olive oil
- green onions, garnish
- 4 tbsp. sour cream, for garnish

Instructions:

Cut florets out of the cauliflower head. In a food processor, pulse cauliflower florets for several seconds till riced and no large bits remain. In a mixing dish, whisk together the eggs using a fork. Combine the cauliflower rice, cheeses, almond flour, salt, garlic powder, and pepper in a mixing bowl. Mix everything together thoroughly, ensuring sure the egg is entirely incorporated. Allow 10 minutes for the mixture to rest. Heat a big nonstick pan over medium heat while the mixture rests. Add the olive oil once the pan is heated. Scoop a quarter cup of the cauliflower fritter batter into the pan. Flatten the fritter mixture with the back of a spatula or the bottom of a 1/4 cup, measuring until it is approximately 1/2 inch thick. The pan can hold roughly 2–3 fritters at a time. Cook for 5–7 minutes on each side before flipping. It's important not to turn the fritters too soon since they're rather delicate while they're first frying. Remove the cooked fritters and lay them on a wire rack to drain any excess oil. As the fritters cool, they will become less delicate and crispier. Serve your fritters with a dollop of sour cream and some chopped green onions as a garnish.

Nutritional Values: Calories: 86 kcal /Carbohydrates: 4 g /Protein: 5 g /Fat: 6 g

Sodium: 72 mg

Chocolate Protein Pancakes

Total Time: 20 mins / **Prep. Time:** 10 mins /**Cooking Time:** 10 mins /**Difficulty:** Easy /**Serving Size:** 2 servings

Ingredients:

- 1 scoop vanilla protein powder
- 1 tbsp. coconut flour
- 1 tbsp. cocoa powder
- 2 tsp. baking powder
- 1 pinch salt
- 1 tbsp. granulated sweetener
- ¼ tsp. vanilla extract
- 4 tbsp. unsalted butter, softened
- 2 eggs
- 1 tbsp. cream cheese

Instructions:

In a mixing dish, combine all the dry ingredients: coconut flour, protein powder, cocoa powder, baking powder, salt, and sweetener until no lumps remain. In the center of the dry ingredients, make a well and add the butter, eggs, vanilla extract, and cream cheese. Leave aside for 5 minutes after gently folding the batter together. Heat a greased nonstick frying pan over medium heat and pour 1/4 cup of batter into the pan. Cook until bubbles appear on the top surface, then turn and cook for an additional 3–4 minutes on the other side. Make pancakes of all the batter by following this method and enjoy.

Nutritional Values: Calories: 379 kcal /Carbohydrates: 5 g /Protein: 19 g /Fat: 31 g

Sodium: 290 mg

Cottage Cheese Breakfast Bowl

Total Time: 10 mins / **Prep. Time:** 10 mins /**Cooking Time:** N/A /**Difficulty:** Easy

Serving Size: 1 serving

Ingredients:

- ½ cup cottage cheese, low fat
- ¼ cup blackberries
- ½ oz. coconut flakes, unsweetened
- ¼ pomegranate
- 1 oz. hazelnuts

Instructions:

Pulse the cottage cheese in a small food processor until it is smooth and creamy, about 2-3 minutes. Remove the pomegranate seeds and prepare the accompanying toppings. Add all the toppings to the blended cheese and give it a good mix. Serve immediately or store in the refrigerator for up to 24 hours.

Nutritional Values: Calories: 226 kcal /Carbohydrates: 19 g /Protein: 18 g /Fat: 14 g

Sodium: 387 mg

Berry Crumble

Total Time: 20 mins / **Prep. Time:** 5 mins /**Cooking Time:** 15 mins /**Difficulty:** Easy /**Serving Size:** 1 serving

Ingredients:

- 1 cup mixed berries
- 1 scoop vanilla protein powder
- 1 tsp. Stevia
- 2 tbsp. lemon juice
- ¼ cup oats
- 10 almonds

Instructions:

Preheat the oven to 350°F. Sprinkle a small amount of Stevia on top of the berries in a small Pyrex baking dish. Combine the oats, protein powder, and lemon juice in a mixing bowl. It'll be rather dry. Mix the chopped almonds with the crumble. On top of the berries, spread the crumble. Bake for 15 minutes, then turn the oven to broil and bake for an additional

1-2 minutes, or until the crumble is slightly brown on top. Remove the dish from the oven and set aside to cool slightly before serving.

Nutritional Values: Calories: 320 kcal /Carbohydrates: 35 g /Protein: 30 g /Fat: 9 g

Sodium: 71 mg

Pumpkin Pancakes

Total Time: 15 mins / **Prep. Time:** 5 mins /**Cooking Time:** 10 mins /**Difficulty:** Easy /**Serving Size:** 3 servings

Ingredients:

- ½ cup oats
- 1 oz. pumpkin puree
- 2 egg whites
- 1 scoop protein powder
- 2 tsp. stevia
- ½ tsp. cinnamon
- Cooking spray
- Apple, for serving
- Sugar-free syrup for serving

Instructions:

In a blender, combine oats, egg whites, pumpkin puree, protein powder, cinnamon, and stevia. Blend until completely smooth. Place a small pan over medium-high heat and coat it with cooking spray. Pour 1/3 of the batter onto the pan and equally distribute it. Allow the pancake to cook for approximately 2 minutes, or until the edges are lightly golden, before turning it and continuing to cook for another 2 minutes. Place the pancake on a platter and put it aside while you finish the other two pancakes. Enjoy with sugar-free syrup and apple slices.

Nutritional Values: Calories: 182 kcal /Carbohydrates: 16 g /Protein: 22 g /Fat: 1 g

Sodium: 218 mg

Bagel With Poached Egg

Total Time: 10 mins / **Prep. Time:** 5 mins /**Cooking Time:** 5 mins /**Difficulty:** Easy

Serving Size: 2 servings

Ingredients:

- 2 bagels
- 1 large tomato
- 2 tbsp. basil pesto

- 2 eggs
- Salt and black pepper to taste
- ¼ Aubergine
- 1 tbsp. olive oil

Instructions:

Tomato and Aubergine should be cut into slices. Each bagel should include 1-2 tomato slices and 1-2 Aubergine slices. Brush the slices with some olive oil, place them on a baking sheet, and roast for 5 minutes at 350°F, flipping once. Poach the two eggs in the pan. Spread 1 tbsp. basil pesto on each bagel. Under the grill, toast the bagels until the edges begin to brown. Place an egg on top of the Aubergine and tomato slices on the bagels. Enjoy!

Nutritional Values: Calories: 361 kcal /Carbohydrates: 38 g /Protein: 17 g /Fat: 4 g

Sodium: 500 mg

Fruity Nutty Muesli

Total Time: 5 mins / **Prep. Time:** 5 mins /**Cooking Time:** N/A /**Difficulty:** Easy

Serving Size: 10 servings

Ingredients:

- 1 pack Muesli Cereal
- ¼ cup sesame seeds
- ½ cup mixed dried fruit
- ½ cup chopped mixed nuts
- ¼ cup sunflower seeds

Instructions:

Combine all of the ingredients in an airtight jar and keep them in a dark cabinet. Serve with yogurt or milk and fresh fruit on top.

Nutritional Values: Calories: 220 kcal /Carbohydrates: 21 g /Protein: 7 g /Fat: 12 g

Sodium: 0 mg

Crunchy Blueberry Yoghurt

Total Time: 5 mins / **Prep. Time:** 5 mins /**Cooking Time:** N/A /**Difficulty:** Easy

Serving Size: 1 serving

Ingredients:

- ¾ cup natural yogurt

- 2 tbsp. muesli
- 3 tbsp. fresh blueberries

Instructions:

Combine all of the ingredients in a bowl and enjoy.

Nutritional Values: Calories: 218 kcal /Carbohydrates: 36 g /Protein: 10 g /Fat: 3 g

Sodium: 100 mg

Strawberry Tofu Smoothie

Total Time: 10 mins / **Prep. Time:** 10 mins /**Cooking Time:** N/A /**Difficulty:** Easy

Serving Size: 2 servings

Ingredients:

- 12 oz. tofu
- 1 cup strawberries, chopped
- 1 tsp. lemon juice
- 2 tbsp. almond butter
- 1 cup almond milk
- ½ cup ice cubes
- 1 tsp. vanilla extract
- 3-5 drops liquid Stevia

Instructions:

All items except the ice cubes should be added to the blender. Blend until completely smooth. Now add the ice cubes and blend until creamy and smooth. Serve immediately with favorite toppings.

Nutritional Values: Calories: 241 kcal /Carbohydrates: 11 g /Protein: 16 g /Fat: 18 g

Sodium: 80 mg

Pineapple Smoothie

Total Time: 5 mins / **Prep. Time:** 5 mins /**Cooking Time:** N/A /**Difficulty:** Easy

Serving Size: 2 servings

Ingredients:

- ¼ cup pineapple chunks
- ½ cup low-fat milk
- ¼ cup natural yogurt
- ¼ cup unsweetened orange juice
- 4 ice cubes

Instructions:

Before using, make sure that all of the ingredients are chilled. Using a hand blender or a smoothie maker, combine the pineapple, milk, yogurt, and juice until

creamy. Add in the ice cubes and blend once more. Fill two glasses with the smoothie and serve.

Nutritional Values: Calories: 89 kcal /Carbohydrates: 16 g /Protein: 3 g /Fat: 1 g

Sodium: 100 mg

Raspberry And Banana Smoothie

Total Time: 5 mins / **Prep. Time:** 5 mins /**Cooking Time:** N/A /**Difficulty:** Easy

Serving Size: 2 servings

Ingredients:

- ¼ cup frozen raspberries
- ½ cup natural yogurt
- 1 medium banana
- 4 ice cubes
- ½ cup low-fat milk
- ½ cup unsweetened orange juice

Instructions:

Before using, make sure that all of the ingredients are chilled. Fruits should be washed and peeled. Using a hand blender or a smoothie maker, combine the fruit, yogurt, milk, and juice until creamy. Add in the ice cubes and blend in the ice cubes once more. Fill two glasses with the smoothie and serve.

Nutritional Values: Calories: 114 kcal /Carbohydrates: 21 g /Protein: 4 g /Fat: 1 g

Sodium: 100 mg

Traditional Porridge

Total Time: 15 mins / **Prep. Time:** 5 mins /**Cooking Time:** 10 mins /**Difficulty:** Easy /**Serving Size:** 1 serving

Ingredients:

- ½ cup dry porridge oats
- 1 tsp. honey
- 1 cup low-fat milk

Instructions:

Put everything in a pot and slowly bring to a boil. Keep a close eye on it since it can quickly boil over. Once it has a boil, reduce the heat to low and continue to cook for 5 to 10 minutes, depending on how mushy you want your oats. Serve with fruits of your choice and enjoy.

Nutritional Values: Calories: 432 kcal /Carbohydrates: 17 g /Protein: 17 g /Fat: 10 g

Sodium: 100 mg

Yogurt, Nut And Banana

Total Time: 5 mins / **Prep. Time:** 5 mins /**Cooking Time:** N/A /**Difficulty:** Easy

Serving Size: 2 servings

Ingredients:

- 1 cup natural yogurt, low-fat
- ½ cup muesli
- 1 tbsp. honey
- 1 ripe banana, chunks
- 3 tbsp. chopped nuts

Instructions:

In the bottom of a bowl, place the banana chunks. Add in the muesli. Pour the yogurt over the top. Add the honey and mix well. Add nuts and give it a mix.

Nutritional Values: Calories: 317 kcal /Carbohydrates: 25 g /Protein: 10 g /Fat: 10 g

Sodium: 100 mg

Parmesan Herb Frittata

Total Time: 30 mins /**Prep. Time:** 10 mins /**Cooking Time:** 20 mins /**Difficulty:** Medium /**Serving Size:** 8 servings

Ingredients:

- 1 tbsp. olive oil
- 1 tbsp. garlic, minced
- ½ onion, diced
- ½ cup milk of choice
- 8 eggs
- ½ tsp. dried oregano
- ¾ tsp. salt
- ¼ tsp. black pepper
- ¼ tsp. cayenne pepper
- 2 tbsp. fresh parsley, chopped
- ¾ cup low-fat mozzarella, shredded
- ½ tsp. dried basil
- 2 roasted red peppers, jarred
- ¾ cup grated parmesan
- ¼ tsp. ground mustard

Instructions:

Preheat the oven to 425°F. On medium-high heat, add olive oil to a cast iron skillet. Once the oil is heated, add the chopped onion. Stir with a spatula while it cooks. Sauté until the onions are nearly tender. Then add the minced garlic to the skillet and sauté for about one minute or until golden. Whisk together the milk, eggs, oregano, salt, cayenne pepper, basil, black pepper, and ground mustard in a separate bowl. Turn off the heat when the garlic and onion are done. Distribute evenly across the bottom of the skillet. Prepare the canned roasted red peppers by dicing them. Spread the red pepper in the skillet as well. On the top layer are parmesan cheese, mozzarella cheese, and fresh parsley. Over everything, pour the egg mixture. Bake it for 16 to 20 minutes, or until the middle is barely set. Check to ensure that the center is not too wiggly before removing it from the oven. Allow a few minutes before serving. While the frittata bubbles vigorously in the oven, it will calm down as it cools.

Nutritional Values: Calories: 167 kcal /Carbohydrates: 3 g /Protein: 12 g /Fat: 12 g

Sodium: 624 mg

Spinach Smoothie

Total Time: 5 mins / **Prep. Time:** 5 mins /**Cooking Time:** N/A /**Difficulty:** Easy

Serving Size: 2 servings

Ingredients:

- 1 cup ice
- 2 tablespoons nut butter of choice
- ½ avocado, pitted
- ½ cup plain Greek yogurt
- 1 tsp. vanilla extract
- 2 cups fresh spinach
- ¼ cup almond milk
- Few drops sweetener

Instructions:

In a blender, combine all of the ingredients, excluding the ice. Blend until completely smooth. Pulse in the ice until it is mostly crushed. Blend the contents until it is thick and creamy. Serve and enjoy.

Nutritional Values: Calories: 236 kcal /Carbohydrates: 11 g /Protein: 11 g /Fat: 16 g

Sodium: 67 mg

Apple Spiced Overnight Oats

Total Time: 2 hours 5 mins / **Prep. Time:** 2 hours 5 mins /**Cooking Time:** N/A /**Difficulty:** Easy /**Serving Size:** 2 servings

Ingredients:

- ¼ cup hemp hearts
- 1 tbsp. chia seeds
- 3 tbsp. rolled oats
- ¼ cup plain Greek yogurt
- 1 tsp. cinnamon
- ¼ cup shredded apple
- 6-8 pecan halves
- ¾ cup milk

Instructions:

Combine the oats, hemp hearts, chia seeds, and cinnamon in a mason jar. Mix the Greek yogurt and shredded apple in the oats. Stir in the milk until everything is completely mixed. Allow the oats to cool in the refrigerator for about 2 hours. Before serving, sprinkle with pecans.

Nutritional Values: Calories: 278 kcal /Carbohydrates: 19 g /Protein: 15 g /Fat: 19 g

Sodium: 13 mg

Sweet Potato Hash

Total Time: 15 mins / **Prep. Time:** 5 mins /**Cooking Time:** 10 mins /**Difficulty:** Medium /**Serving Size:** 4 servings

Ingredients:

- 2 large sweet potatoes, cubes
- 1 small bell pepper, chopped
- 2 tbsp. olive oil
- ½ tsp. kosher salt
- 1 tsp. smoked paprika
- 5 scallions, thinly sliced
- 1 tbsp. pickled jalapeños, chopped
- 1 tbsp. fresh parsley, chopped

Instructions:

In a microwave-safe dish, combine 2 tbsp. of water with the sweet potatoes. Cover and microwave on high for about 10 minutes, or until fork-tender sweet potatoes. In a large skillet, heat the oil over medium-high heat. Add the sweet potatoes, smoked paprika, bell pepper, and salt once the pan is heated. Cook, occasionally stirring, for approximately 5 minutes, or until the sweet potatoes have browned. Cook for another 2 minutes after adding the pickled jalapenos and scallions. Garnish with fresh parsley and divide among 4 serving dishes.

Nutritional Values: Calories: 225 kcal /Carbohydrates: 39 g /Protein: 4 g /Fat: 7 g

Sodium: 248 mg

Chapter 7: Lunch Recipes

Lunch is an important meal of your day. It gives you enough minerals and energy to keep your brain and body running smoothly throughout day. A home-made lunch is a delicious and healthy option that allows you to choose the components of your food. Different types of food and providing the appropriate balance of foods which give you the nutrients your body requires to stay fit and healthy are the keys to a healthy lunch.

In this chapter, you'll find several healthy and delicious lunch choices for people with type-2 diabetes.

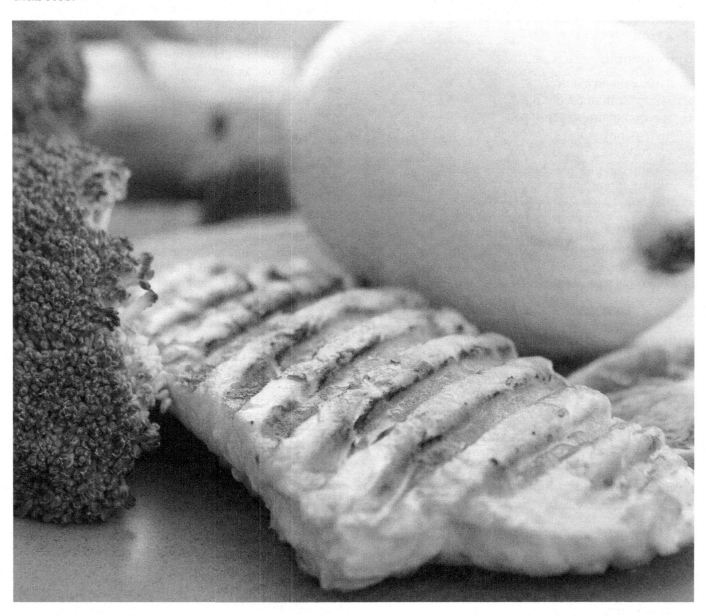

Salmon Chopped Salad

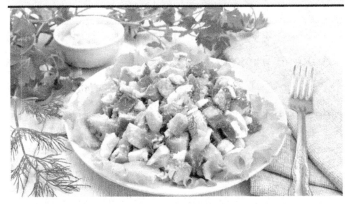

Total Time: 22 mins / **Prep. Time:** 10 mins
/**Cooking Time:** 12 mins /**Difficulty:** Easy
/**Serving Size:** 4 servings

Ingredients:

- 6 oz. cooked salmon
- 3 cups tomatoes, chopped
- 3 cups cucumber, chopped
- 2 tbsp. olive oil
- ½ cup green onions, chopped
- ¾ cup red onions, chopped
- 1 tbsp. lemon juice
- Salt and black pepper to taste

Instructions:

Combine the cucumber, salmon, red onions, tomatoes, and green onions in a large salad bowl. Pour the olive oil and lemon juice into a mason jar. Season with salt and pepper and mix everything together and then pour over the salad. Enjoy.

Nutritional Values: Calories: 166 kcal
/Carbohydrates: 11 g /

Protein: 10 g /Fat: 10 g/Sodium: 321 mg

Skillet Chicken Tenders

Total Time: 24 mins / **Prep. Time:** 10 mins
/**Cooking Time:** 14 mins /**Difficulty:** Easy
/**Serving Size:** 4 servings

Ingredients:

- 1½ lb. chicken tenders
- 1 tsp. rotisserie seasoning
- 2 tbsp. Bbq sauce
- 1 tbsp. olive oil

Instructions:

In a plastic bag, combine all ingredients except the

olive oil. Allow to marinate in the refrigerator. In a medium to large iron skillet, heat the olive oil over medium heat. In a pan, brown the chicken tenders until they are thoroughly cooked. For even browning, turn regularly.

Nutritional Values: Calories: 240 kcal
/Carbohydrates: 3 g /

Protein: 36 g /Fat: 7 g/Sodium: 337 mg

Stuffed Potato

Total Time: 15 mins / **Prep. Time:** 10 mins
/**Cooking Time:** 5 mins /**Difficulty:**
Easy/**Serving Size:** 3 servings

Ingredients:

- 8 oz. baked potato skin on
- 6 oz. grilled chicken tenders
- 2 cups broccoli, steamed
- ¼ cup grated cheddar cheese
- 1 tbsp. diced green onions
- 2 tbsp. BBQ sauce, low sugar
- ½ cup sour cream

Instructions:

Slice the potato in half in an oven-safe pan, then crosswise several times to produce tiny bits. Potato pieces should be equally distributed throughout the skillet. Chicken tenders, Broccoli, and Bbq sauce go on top of the potato. Cheese should be sprinkled on top. To melt the cheese, place the potato under the broiler. Sour cream and green onion go on top. Divide the mixture into three parts and serve.

Nutritional Values: Calories: 397 kcal
/Carbohydrates: 15 g /

Protein: 36 g /Fat: 20 g/Sodium: 334 mg

Tuna Nicoise Salad

Total Time: 15 mins / **Prep. Time:** 10 mins
/**Cooking Time:** 5 mins /**Difficulty:** Medium
/**Serving Size:** 4 serving

Ingredients:

- 4 oz. ahi tuna steak
- 2 cups baby spinach
- 1 whole egg
- 1 cup broccoli
- 1 ½ cup green beans
- 2 cucumbers
- ½ cup red bell pepper
- 3 large black olives

- 1 radish
- 1 tsp. olive oil
- Handful of parsley
- ½ tsp. Dijon mustard
- 1 tsp. balsamic vinegar
- ½ tsp. pepper

Instructions:

Boil the egg for 12 minutes in boiling hot water and then set it aside to cool. Steam the broccoli and beans. It just takes 3 minutes in a saucepan of boiling water or 2-3 minutes in the microwave with a little water. In a large skillet, heat a little oil over high heat. Season the tuna on all sides with pepper, then put it in the pan and cook for 2 minutes on each side. Place the spinach in a salad bowl or on a dish. The cucumber, bell pepper, and boiled egg should all be cut into bite-size pieces. On top of the spinach, sprinkle a pinch of salt and pepper. Slice the radish and combine it with the steamed beans and broccoli, and olives in a mixing bowl. Toss them with the spinach salad. Toss in the tuna slices in the salad. Combine the balsamic vinegar, olive oil, salt, mustard, and pepper in a mixing bowl. Add chopped parsley to the salad dressing and drizzle the prepared salad dressing all over the salad with a spoon. Serve and enjoy.

Nutritional Values: Calories: 405 kcal /Carbohydrates: 18 g /

Protein: 39 g /Fat: 13 g/Sodium: 586 mg

Chicken Philly Cheesesteak

Total Time: 25 mins / **Prep. Time:** 10 mins /**Cooking Time:** 15 mins /**Difficulty:** Medium /**Serving Size:** 3 servings

Ingredients:

- 10 oz. boneless chicken breasts
- ½ tsp. onion powder
- 2 tbsp. Worcestershire sauce
- 2 tsp. olive oil, divided
- ½ tsp. garlic powder
- ½ cup diced onion
- 1 dash ground pepper
- ½ tsp. minced garlic
- ½ cup diced bell pepper
- 3 slices provolone cheese

Instructions:

Place chicken breasts on chopping board and slice

into very thin slices. Add sliced chicken to a mixing bowl and stir in the Worcestershire sauce, garlic powder, onion powder and ground pepper to coat the chicken. In a large oven-safe skillet, heat 1 teaspoon tsp. olive oil. Cook until the chicken pieces are browned, about 5 minutes. Cook for another 2-3 minutes or until brown on the other side. Remove the pan from the heat. In the same skillet, add the remaining 1 tsp. olive oil. After that, toss in the bell pepper, onions, and garlic. Cook for 2-3 minutes, stirring occasionally, until heated and tender. Turn off the heat and return the chicken to the skillet with the vegetables, stirring to incorporate. Cover with sliced cheese and let aside for 2-3 minutes to melt.

Nutritional Values: Calories: 263 kcal /Carbohydrates: 5 g /

Protein: 27 g /Fat: 13 g/Sodium: 330 mg

Chicken, Cabbage and Peach Salad

Total Time: 10 mins / **Prep. Time:** 10 mins /**Cooking Time:** N/A /**Difficulty:** Easy

Serving Size: 3 servings

Ingredients:

- 1½ cups cooked chicken breast, diced
- 1 medium ripe peach, diced
- 1 cup red cabbage, shredded
- ¼ cup plain yogurt, fat-free
- 1 stalk celery, diced
- ¼ tsp. curry powder
- 1/8 tsp. salt
- 3 tbsp. peach nectar
- 1/8 tsp. black pepper

Instructions:

In a medium mixing bowl, combine the cabbage, chicken, peach, and celery. Toss lightly but thoroughly. In a small bowl, combine the peach nectar, yogurt, salt, curry powder and pepper. Toss the dressing with salad. Mix gently but thoroughly.

Nutritional Values: Calories: 154 kcal /Carbohydrates: 10 g /

Protein: 23 g /Fat: 2 g/Sodium: 174 mg

Cauliflower Potato Salad

Total Time: 25 mins / **Prep. Time:** 10 mins /**Cooking Time:** 15 mins /**Difficulty:** Easy /**Serving Size:** 4 servings

Ingredients:

- ¼ cup red onion, chopped
- 5 cups cauliflower florets
- 1/3 cup celery, chopped
- ½ yellow bell pepper, chopped
- 2 hard-boiled eggs, chopped
- ¼ cup mayonnaise
- 1 tsp. apple cider vinegar
- 1 tsp. yellow mustard
- Salt and pepper, to taste
- ½ tsp. garlic, minced
- ½ tsp. paprika
- Fresh parsley, chopped

Instructions:

Fill a big saucepan with around 2 cups of water and a steamer basket to steam the flowers of cauliflower. Bring the water to a boil and f ill the steamer basket halfway with cauliflower florets. Cover and steam till the cauliflower florets is fork tender, about 15 minutes. Remove the steamed cauliflower florets from the heat and set aside to cool for 5 minutes. In a mixing dish, combine the steamed cauliflower, red onion, yellow bell pepper, celery, and hard-boiled eggs. To make the dressing, combine mayonnaise, apple cider vinegar, mustard, salt and pepper in a small bowl and whisk to blend. Check for seasoning before pouring the dressing over the salad. Mix the salad with dressing in a large mixing bowl and stir until thoroughly blended. Fresh chopped parsley and paprika are sprinkled over top. Serve and enjoy.

Nutritional Values: Calories: 117 kcal /Carbohydrates: 6 g /

Protein: 4 g /Fat: 9 g/Sodium: 317 mg

Hamburger Vegetable Soup

Total Time: 40 mins / **Prep. Time:** 10 mins /**Cooking Time:** 30 mins /**Difficulty:** Easy /**Serving Size:** 6 servings

Ingredients:

- ½ lb. ground beef
- 14.5 oz. canned tomatoes, diced
- 32 oz. beef broth, low- sodium
- 1 cup sliced carrots
- 14.5 oz. canned green beans
- ¾ cup cooked pasta
- ¾ cup corn
- 2 tbsp. ketchup
- 1 tbsp. Worcestershire sauce
- 1 tsp. thyme, crushed
- ½ tsp. salt

Instructions:

Brown the ground beef in a medium soup pot over medium heat. Mix together the remaining ingredients. Cook for 30 minutes. Seasonings can be adjusted as needed.

Nutritional Values: Calories: 207 kcal /Carbohydrates: 20 g /

Protein: 13 g /Fat: 8 g/Sodium: 685 mg

Tomato Pie

Total Time: 40 mins / **Prep. Time:** 10 mins /**Cooking Time:** 30 mins /**Difficulty:** Medium /**Serving Size:** 4 servings

Ingredients:

- ½ prepared pie crust
- 1/3 cup green onion, chopped
- 1 large tomato, sliced
- 1 cup cheese, grated
- 10 basil leaves, chopped
- 1/8 tsp. salt
- ¼ cup mayo
- dash ground pepper

Instructions:

Using cutter cut a prepared roll of pie crust in half. Return the unused 1/2 to the refrigerator to be used later. Roll out the remaining 1/2 crust thinly and fit into an 8" pan after gently flouring the top. Bake the crust for 10 minutes at 350°F, or until gently browned, after pricking with a fork. Meanwhile, gently salt the sliced tomatoes and drain them in a strainer or on paper towels. In a prebaked crust, layer green onions, drained tomatoes, and basil. Combine the cheese, mayonnaise, salt, and pepper in a small bowl. On top of the basil, spread the mixture. Bake for 20 minutes at 350°F, or until bubbling and cheese begins to brown.

Nutritional Values: Calories: 317 kcal /Carbohydrates: 13 g /

Protein: 9 g /Fat: 25 g/Sodium: 428 mg

Turkey Roll-Up

Total Time: 5 mins / **Prep. Time:** 5 mins /**Cooking Time:** N/A /**Difficulty:** Easy

Serving Size: 1 serving

Ingredients:

- 1 low carb tortilla wrap
- 2 oz. roasted turkey
- 1 tbsp. low carb honey mustard
- 1 slice cheese
- lettuce leaf
- ½ diced tomato

Instructions:

Spread honey mustard over a wrap and place it on wax paper or foil. Fill the wrap with the remaining ingredients and roll it up. If desired, cut the wrap in half.

Nutritional Values: Calories: 242 kcal /Carbohydrates: 4 g /

Protein: 15 g /Fat: 17 g/Sodium: 323 mg

Rotisserie Chicken

Total Time: 55 mins / **Prep. Time:** 10 mins /**Cooking Time:** 45 mins /**Difficulty:** Easy /**Serving Size:** 8 servings

Ingredients:

2½ lb. chicken pieces

1 tbsp. Rotisserie Seasoning

Instructions:

Preheat the oven to 375°F. Place the chicken on a metal baking pan lined with foil or parchment paper. Rotisserie seasoning should be applied to both sides of the chicken pieces. Roast the chicken for 45 minutes, or until chicken is thoroughly cooked.

Nutritional Values: Calories: 310 kcal /Carbohydrates: 1 g /

Protein: 27 g /Fat: 21 g/Sodium: 100 mg

Pork Tacos With Mango Salsa

Total Time: 30 mins / **Prep. Time:** 25 mins /**Cooking Time:** 5 mins /**Difficulty:** Medium /**Serving Size:** 12 servings

Ingredients:

- 2 tbsp. lime juice
- 2 tbsp. white vinegar
- 1 small red onion, coarsely chopped
- 3 cups cubed fresh pineapple
- 2 chipotle peppers in adobo sauce
- 3 tbsp. chili powder
- 1½ tsp. salt
- 2 tsp. ground cumin
- ½ tsp. pepper
- 3 lbs. pork tenderloin, cubes
- 12 oz. dark Mexican beer
- 16 oz. mango salsa
- ¼ cup fresh cilantro, chopped
- Optional toppings: cubed avocado Cubed fresh pineapple, and queso fresco
- 24 corn tortillas, warmed

Instructions:

In a blender, puree the first nine ingredients; whisk in the beer. Combine the meat and pineapple mixture in a 6-quart electric pressure cooker. Close the pressure-release valve and lock the lid. Adjust to high pressure and cook for 3 minutes. Release the pressure. A thermometer put into the pork should register a temperature of at least 145°F. To break up the meat, stir it around. Toss the cilantro into the salsa. Divide pork mixture in tortillas using a slotted spoon; serve with salsa and garnishes as desired.

Nutritional Values: Calories: 284 kcal /Carbohydrates: 30 g /

Protein: 26 g /Fat: 6 g/Sodium: 678 mg

Chicken With Peach-Avocado Salsa

Total Time: 30 mins / **Prep. Time:** 15 mins /**Cooking Time:** 15 mins /**Difficulty:** Easy /**Serving Size:** 4 servings

Ingredients:

- 1 peach, peeled and chopped
- ½ cup sweet red pepper, chopped
- 1 avocado, peeled and cubed
- 1 tbsp. fresh basil, minced
- 3 tbsp. red onion, finely chopped
- 1 tsp. hot pepper sauce
- 1 tbsp. lime juice
- ¾ tsp. salt, divided
- ½ tsp. grated lime zest
- 4 skinless chicken breast halves

- ½ tsp. pepper, divided

Instructions:

Combine avocado, peaches, onion, red pepper, lime juice, basil, lime zest, hot sauce, 1/4 tsp. salt, and 1/4 tsp. pepper in a small bowl for salsa. Add the remaining pepper and salt to the chicken. Grill chicken for 5 minutes, covered, on a lightly oiled grill rack over medium heat. Turn and cook for another 7-9 minutes, or until a thermometer reads 165°. Serve with a side of salsa.

Nutritional Values: Calories: 265 kcal /Carbohydrates: 9 g /

Protein: 36 g /Fat: 9 g/Sodium: 536 mg

Chicken And Spanish Cauliflower Rice

Total Time: 28 mins / **Prep. Time:** 10 mins /**Cooking Time:** 18 mins /**Difficulty:** Medium/**Serving Size:** 4 servings

Ingredients:

- 1 large head cauliflower
- ½ tsp. salt
- 1 lb. skinless chicken breasts, cubes
- 1 tbsp. canola oil
- ½ tsp. pepper
- 1 small onion, chopped
- 1 medium green pepper, chopped
- ½ cup tomato juice
- 1 garlic clove, minced
- ¼ cup fresh cilantro, chopped
- ¼ tsp. ground cumin
- 1 tbsp. lime juice

Instructions:

Cauliflower should be cored and chopped into 1-inch pieces. In a food processor, pulse cauliflower in batches until it resembles rice. Season the chicken cubes with salt and pepper before serving. Heat the oil in a large pan over medium-high heat and cook the chicken until it is nicely browned, around 5 minutes. Cook and stir for 3 minutes after adding the green pepper, garlic and onion. Bring to a boil, stirring in the tomato juice and cumin. Simmer, covered, over medium heat for 7-10 minutes, or until cauliflower is cooked, stirring occasionally. Add the lime juice and cilantro and mix well.

Nutritional Values: Calories: 227 kcal /Carbohydrates: 15 g /

Protein: 28 g /Fat: 7 g/Sodium: 492 mg

Grilled Chicken Chopped Salad

Total Time: 30 mins / **Prep. Time:** 15 mins /**Cooking Time:** 15 mins /**Difficulty:** Medium/**Serving Size:** 4 servings

Ingredients:

- 1 lb. chicken tenderloins
- 2 zucchini, quartered lengthwise
- 6 tbsp. Italian salad dressing, divided
- 2 ears sweet corn, husked
- 1 red onion, quartered
- 1 medium cucumber, chopped
- 1 bunch romaine, chopped

Instructions:

Toss the chicken with 4 tbsp. of the dressing in a mixing bowl. Brush the remaining 2 tbsp. of dressing over the zucchini and onion. Place the corn, onion and zucchini on a grill rack over medium heat and close the lid. Grill the zucchini and onions for 2-3 minutes on each side, or until they are soft. Grill corn for 10-12 minutes, turning once or twice, until tender. Drain the chicken and toss out the marinade. Cover and grill the chicken for 3-4 minutes per side over medium heat, or until no longer pink. Remove the corn off the cobs and chop the zucchini, onion, and chicken into bite-size pieces. Layer cucumber, romaine, grilled vegetables, and chicken in a 3-quart trifle dish or other glass bowl. Serve with extra dressing if desired.

Nutritional Values: Calories: 239 kcal /Carbohydrates: 21 g /

Protein: 32 g /Fat: 5 g/Sodium: 276 mg

Fish Tacos With Berry Salsa

Total Time: 15 mins / **Prep. Time:** 10 mins /**Cooking Time:** 5 mins /**Difficulty:** Easy /**Serving Size:** 4 servings

Ingredients:

- 1 cup peeled jicama, chopped
- 1 jalapeno pepper, finely chopped
- 1 cup fresh strawberries, chopped
- 2 tbsp. lime juice

- 3 tbsp. fresh cilantro, minced
- ½ tsp. salt, divided
- ¼ tsp. pepper
- 4 tilapia fillets
- ½ cup Cotija cheese, crumbled
- 8 corn tortillas

Instructions:

Preheat the oven to broil. To make the salsa, put the first five ingredients in a small dish and season with 1/4 tsp. salt. Sprinkle pepper and the remaining salt over the fillets in a foil-lined baking pan. Broil 5-7 minutes, 4-6 inches from heat or until salmon flakes easily with a fork. Serve the fish with cheese and salsa in tortillas.

Nutritional Values: Calories: 329 kcal /Carbohydrates: 29 g /

Protein: 38 g /Fat: 8 g/Sodium: 599 mg

Chicken With Tomatoes

Total Time: 25 mins / **Prep. Time:** 10 mins /**Cooking Time:** 15 mins /**Difficulty:** Medium/**Serving Size:** 4 servings

Ingredients:

- 2 tbsp. garlic herb seasoning blend, salt-free
- ¼ tsp. Italian seasoning
- ½ tsp. salt
- 1/8 tsp. red pepper flakes, optional
- ¼ tsp. pepper
- 1 tbsp. olive oil
- 4 skinless, chicken breast halves
- ¾ lb. fresh green beans, trimmed
- 14 oz. fire-roasted diced tomatoes, undrained
- 1 tbsp. butter
- 2 tbsp. water

Instructions:

Combine the seasoning ingredients and season both sides of the chicken breasts. Heat the oil in a large skillet over medium heat. Both sides of the chicken should be browned. Bring to a boil with the tomatoes. Reduce heat to low; cover and cook for 10-12 minutes. Meanwhile, mix green beans and water in a 2-quart microwave-safe dish; microwave on high for 3-4 minutes or until tender. Drain. Remove the chicken from the skillet and set it aside to remain warm. Toss the tomato combination with the butter and beans and serve with chicken.

Nutritional Values: Calories: 294 kcal /Carbohydrates: 12 g /

Protein: 37 g /Fat: 12 g/Sodium: 681 mg

Fish Tacos

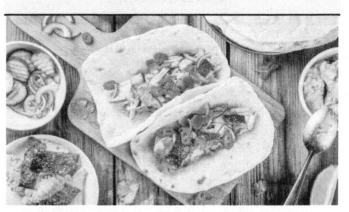

Total Time: 18 mins / **Prep. Time:** 10 mins /**Cooking Time:** 8 mins /**Difficulty:** Easy /**Serving Size:** 2 servings

Ingredients:

- 1 tsp. seeded jalapeno pepper, chopped
- 1 cup coleslaw mix
- 1 green onion, sliced
- ¼ cup fresh cilantro, chopped
- 4 tsp. canola oil, divided
- ½ tsp. ground cumin
- ½ tsp. salt, divided
- 2 tsp. lime juice
- 2 tilapia fillets
- ¼ tsp. pepper, divided
- ½ ripe avocado, peeled and sliced

Instructions:

Toss the first four ingredients with 2 tsp. oil, cumin, lime juice, 1/4 tsp. salt, and 1/8 tsp. pepper in a mixing bowl. Refrigerate until ready to serve. Using paper towels pat the fillets dry and season with the leftover salt and pepper. Cook tilapia in remaining oil in a large nonstick pan over medium-high heat until it just begins to flake effortlessly with a fork, 3-4 minutes each side. Serve with avocado and slaw on top.

Nutritional Values: Calories: 293 kcal /Carbohydrates: 6 g /

Protein: 33 g /Fat: 16 g/Sodium: 663 mg

Sesame Chicken with Couscous

Total Time: 30 mins / **Prep. Time:** 15 mins /**Cooking Time:** 15 mins /**Difficulty:** Medium/**Serving Size:** 4 servings

Ingredients:

- 1½ cups water
- 1 tbsp. olive oil
- 1 cup whole wheat couscous, uncooked
- 4 green onions, sliced
- 2 cups coleslaw mix
- 2 cups cooked chicken breast, shredded
- 2 tbsp. + ½ cup low-fat sesame salad dressing, divided
- Chopped peanuts, optional
- 2 tbsp. fresh cilantro, minced

Instructions:

Bring water to a boil in a small saucepan. Toss in the couscous. Remove from heat and let aside for 5-10 minutes, covered, until water has been absorbed. Using a fork, fluff the mixture. Heat the oil in a large nonstick skillet over medium heat. Cook and stir for 3-4 minutes, or just until the coleslaw mix is tender. Mix and cook the green onions, 2 tbsp. dressing, and couscous. Remove couscous from pan and set aside to keep warm. Add the chicken and the remaining 1/2 cup dressing to the same skillet and cook and mix over medium heat until cooked through. Serve over couscous with cilantro and peanuts, if preferred.

Nutritional Values: Calories: 320 kcal /Carbohydrates: 35 g /

Protein: 26 g /Fat: 9 g/Sodium: 442 mg

Grilled Chicken and Greens

Total Time: 25 mins / **Prep. Time:** 13 mins /**Cooking Time:** 12 mins /**Difficulty:** Medium /**Serving Size:** 4 servings

Ingredients:

- 6 garlic cloves, minced
- ¼ cup orange juice
- 1½ tsp. dried thyme
- 1 tbsp. balsamic vinegar
- ½ tsp. salt
- 4 skinless chicken breast halves

- 2 cups cherry tomatoes, halved
- 10 oz. spring mix salad greens
- ¼ cup pitted Greek olives, halved
- ½ cup feta cheese, crumbled
- ¼ cup prepared vinaigrette

Instructions:

Add the first five ingredients in a large resealable plastic bag. Seal the bag and flip the chicken to coat it. Refrigerate for 8 hours or overnight in the refrigerator. Drain the chicken and toss out the marinade. Soak a paper towel with cooking oil and rub it on the grill rack with long-handled tongs to gently coat it. 5-6 minutes on each side, over medium heat or grill 4 in. from flame. Combine the greens, tomatoes, feta cheese, and olives in a large mixing dish. Drizzle vinaigrette over salad and toss to coat. Serve with salad and sliced chicken.

Nutritional Values: Calories: 282 kcal /Carbohydrates: 12 g /

Protein: 33 g /Fat: 11 g/Sodium: 717 mg

Sesame Turkey Stir-Fry

Total Time: 20 mins / **Prep. Time:** 10 mins /**Cooking Time:** 10 mins /**Difficulty:** Medium /**Serving Size:** 4 servings

Ingredients:

- 1/8 tsp. red pepper flakes
- 1 tsp. cornstarch
- 2 tbsp. low-sodium soy sauce
- ½ cup water
- 2 tsp. curry powder
- 1 tbsp. honey
- 2 tsp. sesame oil
- 1 onion, sliced into thin wedges
- 1 sweet red pepper, julienned
- 2 cups cooked turkey breast, shredded
- 1 garlic clove, minced
- 2 cups hot cooked brown rice
- 1 green onion, sliced
- toasted sesame seeds, for garnish
- sliced serrano pepper, for garnish

Instructions:

Combine the first six ingredients in a small bowl until well combined. Heat the oil in a large skillet over medium-high heat. Stir in the onion and red pepper until crisp-tender. Cook for a further minute after adding the garlic. Add the cornstarch mixture to the pan and stir well. Bring to a boil, then reduce to a low heat and simmer for 2 minutes, or until the sauce has thickened. Heat the turkey until it is fully cooked. Add the green onion and mix well. Serve with a side of rice. Top with sesame seeds and serrano pepper and serve.

Nutritional Values: Calories: 269 kcal /Carbohydrates: 32 g /

Protein: 25 g /Fat: 4 g/Sodium: 349 mg

Grilled Steak with Salad

Total Time: 35 mins / **Prep. Time:** 20 mins /**Cooking Time:** 15 mins /**Difficulty:** Medium/**Serving Size:** 4 servings

Ingredients:

- 1½ lb. beef top sirloin steak
- 3 tsp. Creole seasoning
- 1 tbsp. olive oil
- 15 oz. cannellini beans, rinsed and drained
- 2 large tomatoes, chopped
- 3 green onions, chopped
- 15 oz. black beans, rinsed and drained
- 2 tsp. grated lemon zest
- ¼ cup minced fresh cilantro
- ¼ tsp. salt
- 2 tbsp. lemon juice
- 1 avocado, cubed

Instructions:

Oil both sides of the steak and season with Creole spice. Grill the steak for 5-8 minutes on each side over medium heat until meat reaches desired doneness. Allow for a 5-minute rest period. Combine tomatoes, green onions, beans, cilantro, lemon juice, lemon zest and salt in a large mixing bowl; gently fold in avocado. Slice the steak and serve with the bean mixture.

Nutritional Values: Calories: 328 kcal /Carbohydrates: 25 g /

Protein: 31 g /Fat: 11 g/Sodium: 710 mg

Summer Garden Fish Tacos

Total Time: 40 mins / **Prep. Time:** 20 mins /**Cooking Time:** 20 mins /**Difficulty:** Medium/**Serving Size:** 4 servings

Ingredients:

- 1 ear sweet corn, husk removed

- 4 tilapia fillets
- 1 poblano pepper, halved
- 1 yellow summer squash, halved lengthwise
- 1/8 tsp. salt
- 1/3 cup red onion, chopped
- 1 medium heirloom tomato, chopped
- 1 tsp. lime zest
- 3 tbsp. fresh cilantro, coarsely chopped
- 8 taco shells, warmed
- 3 tbsp. lime juice
- ½ ripe avocado, peeled and sliced

Instructions:

Brush the grill rack with a little coating of oil. Cover and grill corn and pepper over medium heat for 10-12 minutes, turning regularly, until tender. Allow to cool slightly. In the meantime, season the fish with salt. Cover and grill the fish and squash over medium heat until the fish flakes easily with a fork and the squash are cooked, about 7-9 minutes, turning once. Remove the corn off the cob and set it in a basin. Pepper and squash should be chopped and added to the corn. Combine the onion, tomato, lime zest, cilantro, and lime juice in a mixing bowl. Top taco shells with fish, corn mixture, and avocado slices.

Nutritional Values: Calories: 278 kcal /Carbohydrates: 26 g /

Protein: 25 g /Fat: 10 g/Sodium: 214 mg

Tuna With White Bean Salad

Total Time: 20 mins / **Prep. Time:** 12 mins /**Cooking Time:** 8 mins /**Difficulty:** Easy /**Serving Size:** 4 servings

Ingredients:

- 15 oz. cannellini beans, rinsed and drained
- 1 red pepper, finely chopped
- 3 celery ribs, finely chopped
- ½ cup fresh basil leaves, thinly sliced
- 1 plum tomato, finely chopped
- ¼ cup red onion, finely chopped
- 2 tbsp. red wine vinegar
- 3 tbsp. + 1 tbsp. olive oil, divided
- ¼ tsp. + ¼ tsp. salt, divided
- 1 tbsp. lemon juice
- 4 tuna steaks
- ¼ tsp. + ¼ tsp. pepper

Instructions:

Add the first 6 ingredients in a large mixing bowl. Whisk together the 3 tbsp. oil, lemon juice, vinegar, 1/4 tsp. salt, and 1/4 tsp. pepper in a small bowl. Toss the bean mixture in the sauce to coat it. Refrigerate until ready to serve. Using a brush, coat the tuna with remaining 1 tbsp. oil. Place on an oiled grill rack and season with salt and pepper. Cook 3-4 minutes on each side, covered, over high heat or 3-4 inches from the fire until slightly pink in the middle for medium-rare. Serve alongside a salad.

Nutritional Values: Calories: 409 kcal /Carbohydrates: 20 g /

Protein: 45 g /Fat: 16 g/Sodium: 517 mg

Chicken and Goat Cheese Skillet

Total Time: 20 mins / **Prep. Time:** 10 mins /**Cooking Time:** 10 mins /**Difficulty:** Medium /**Serving Size:** 2 servings

Ingredients:

- ½ lb. skinless chicken breasts, 1-inch pieces
- 1/8 tsp. pepper
- ¼ tsp. salt
- 1 cup fresh asparagus, 1-inch pieces
- 2 tsp. olive oil
- 3 tbsp. 2% milk
- 3 plum tomatoes, chopped
- 1 garlic clove, minced
- 2 tbsp. herbed fresh goat cheese, crumbled

Instructions:

Season the chicken with salt and pepper. Heat oil in a large pan over medium-high heat and cook chicken till no longer pink, about 4-6 minutes. Remove from the pan and set aside. Cook and stir asparagus in skillet for 1 minute over medium-high heat. Cook and stir for 30 seconds after adding the garlic. Add the remaining ingredients and cook over medium heat until milk, tomatoes, and added cheese begin to melt, about 2-3 minutes. Add the chicken and mix well.

Nutritional Values: Calories: 251 kcal /Carbohydrates: 8 g /

Protein: 29 g /Fat: 11 g/Sodium: 447 mg

Shrimp Orzo with Feta

Total Time: 25 mins / **Prep. Time:** 15 mins /**Cooking Time:** 10 mins /**Difficulty:** Medium/**Serving Size:** 4 servings

Ingredients:

- 1¼ cups whole wheat orzo pasta, uncooked
- 2 garlic cloves, minced
- 2 tbsp. olive oil
- 2 tbsp. lemon juice
- 2 medium tomatoes, chopped
- 2 tbsp. fresh cilantro, minced
- 1¼ lb. uncooked shrimp, peeled and deveined
- ½ cup feta cheese, crumbled
- ¼ tsp. pepper

Instructions:

Cook orzo as directed on the packet. Meanwhile heat the oil in a large pan over medium heat. Add garlic to the pan and cook for 1 minute, stirring constantly. Toss in the tomatoes and the lemon juice. Bring it to a boil and add the shrimp and mix well. Reduce heat to low and cook, uncovered, for 4-5 minutes, or until shrimp become pink. Orzo should be drained. Stir through the orzo, cilantro, and pepper in the shrimp mixture. Feta cheese should be sprinkled on top.

Nutritional Values: Calories: 406 kcal /Carbohydrates: 40 g /

Protein: 33 g /Fat: 12 g/Sodium: 307 mg

Savory Braised Chicken

Total Time: 55 mins / **Prep. Time:** 15 mins /**Cooking Time:** 40 mins /**Difficulty:** Medium/**Serving Size:** 6 servings

Ingredients:

- ½ cup seasoned bread crumbs
- 2 tbsp. olive oil
- 6 skinless chicken breast halves
- 2 tbsp. tomato paste
- 14 oz. beef broth
- ½ tsp. salt
- 1 tsp. poultry seasoning
- 1 lb. fresh baby carrots
- ½ tsp. pepper
- 2 medium zucchini, sliced
- 1 lb. fresh mushrooms, sliced

Instructions:

In a small dish, put the bread crumbs. Coat both sides of the chicken breasts with bread crumbs and brush off excess. Heat the oil in a Dutch oven over medium heat. Cook the coated chicken breasts for 2-4 minutes each side or until browned in batches. Take the chicken out of the pan. In the same pan, combine tomato paste, broth, and spices; simmer over medium-high heat, swirling to release browned pieces from the bottom of the pan. Add the vegetables to the pan and bring the veggies and chicken to a boil. Reduce to a low heat and cook, covered, for 25-30 minutes, or until veggies are tender.

Nutritional Values: Calories: 247 kcal /Carbohydrates: 16 g /

Protein: 28 g /Fat: 8 g/Sodium: 703 mg

Garlic Tilapia

Total Time: 13 mins / **Prep. Time:** 5 mins /**Cooking Time:** 8 mins /**Difficulty:** Easy

Serving Size: 4 servings

Ingredients:

- 4 tilapia fillets
- ½ tsp. garlic salt
- ¼ tsp. pepper
- 1 tbsp. olive oil

Instructions:

Season the fish with pepper and garlic salt. Heat the oil in a large skillet over medium heat. Cook the tilapia for 3-4 minutes on each side, or until it flakes easily with a fork.

Nutritional Values: Calories: 300 kcal /Carbohydrates: 15 g /

Protein: 29 g /Fat: 5 g/Sodium: 550 mg

Chicken Tacos with Avocado Salsa

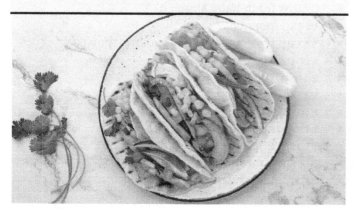

Total Time: 20 mins / **Prep. Time:** 10 mins /**Cooking Time:** 10 mins /**Difficulty:** Medium/**Serving Size:** 4 servings

Ingredients:

- 1/3 cup water

- 1 lb. skinless chicken breasts strips
- 1 tsp. onion powder
- 1 tbsp. chili powder
- 1 tsp. ground cumin
- 1 tsp. dried oregano
- ½ tsp. salt
- 1 tsp. paprika
- ½ tsp. garlic powder
- 1 cup corn
- 1 ripe avocado, peeled and cubed
- 2 tsp. lime juice
- 1 cup cherry tomatoes, quartered
- 8 taco shells, warmed

Instructions:

Over medium-high heat, coat a large skillet with cooking spray and brown the chicken been browned. Combine the water and spices in the skillet and cook tossing periodically, for 4-5 minutes or till chicken is no longer pink. Meanwhile, carefully combine corn, avocado, tomatoes, and lime juice in a small bowl. Fill taco shells with chicken mixture and avocado salsa.

Nutritional Values: Calories: 354 kcal /Carbohydrates: 30 g /

Protein: 27 g /Fat: 15 g/Sodium: 474 mg

Healthy Tuscan Chicken

Total Time: 40 mins / **Prep. Time:** 25 mins /**Cooking Time:** 15 mins /**Difficulty:** Medium/**Serving Size:** 4 servings

Ingredients:

- 4 skinless chicken breast halves
- 2 tbsp. olive oil
- ¼ tsp. pepper
- 1 red pepper, julienned
- 1 yellow pepper, julienned
- 1 green pepper, julienned
- 2 garlic cloves, minced
- 2 thin slices prosciutto, chopped
- ¼ cup low-sodium chicken broth
- 14 oz. diced tomatoes, undrained
- 1 tsp. fresh oregano, minced
- 2 tbsp. fresh basil, minced

Instructions:

Season the chicken with salt and pepper. Brown the chicken in oil in a large nonstick pan. Remove from the pan and keep warm. Sauté the peppers and prosciutto in the same pan until the peppers are soft. Cook for a further minute after adding the garlic. Toss in the broth, tomatoes, basil, and oregano, as well as the chicken. Bring the broth to a boil. Reduce to a low heat, cover, and cook for 12-15 minutes.

Nutritional Values: Calories: 304 kcal /Carbohydrates: 11 g /

Protein: 38 g /Fat: 12 g/Sodium: 389 mg

Spicy Turkey Tenderloin

Total Time: 45 mins / **Prep. Time:** 20 mins /**Cooking Time:** 25 mins /**Difficulty:** Medium/**Serving Size:** 2 servings

Ingredients:

- ½ tsp. chili powder
- ¼ tsp. salt
- ½ tsp. ground cumin
- ½ lb. turkey breast tenderloin
- 1/8 tsp. cayenne pepper
- ¼ cup chicken broth
- 2 tsp. olive oil
- 2 tbsp. lime juice

Instructions:

Combine the cumin, chilli powder, salt, and cayenne in a small bowl. Spice mixture should be sprinkled over the turkey. Brown the turkey in a pan with 2 tsp. oil for 3-4 minutes on each side. In a skillet, combine the broth and lime juice. Reduce heat to low, cover, and cook for 15-18 minutes, or until turkey juices run transparent.

Nutritional Values: Calories: 342 kcal /Carbohydrates: 32 g /

Protein: 35 g /Fat: 9 g/Sodium: 767 mg

Artichoke Ratatouille Chicken

Total Time: 1 hour 25 mins / **Prep. Time:** 25 mins /**Cooking Time:** 1 hour /**Difficulty:** Easy /**Serving Size:** 6 servings

Ingredients:

- 1 lb. Japanese eggplants
- 1 sweet yellow pepper
- 4 plum tomatoes
- 1 medium onion
- 1 sweet red pepper
- 2 tbsp. minced fresh thyme
- 14 oz. artichoke hearts, drained and quartered
- 2 tbsp. olive oil

- 2 tbsp. capers, drained
- 1 tsp. Creole seasoning, divided
- 2 garlic cloves, minced
- 1 cup white wine
- 1½ lb. skinless chicken breasts, cubed
- ¼ cup grated Asiago cheese

Instructions:

Transfer tomatoes, eggplants, onion and peppers to a large mixing bowl and cut into 3/4-inch pieces. Add 1/2 tsp. Creole seasoning, artichoke hearts, capers, thyme, oil, garlic Season the chicken with the rest of the Creole spice. Place the chicken in a 13x9-inch baking dish covered with cooking spray, and top with the vegetable mixture. Pour wine over the veggies. Preheat oven to 350°F and bake for 30 minutes, covered. Uncover and bake for another 30-45 minutes, or until the chicken is no longer pink and the veggies are soft. Cheese should be sprinkled on top.

Nutritional Values: Calories: 252 kcal /Carbohydrates: 15 g /

Protein: 28 g /Fat: 9 g/Sodium: 468 mg

Grilled Tuna with Greens

Total Time: 0 mins / **Prep. Time:** 0 mins /**Cooking Time:** 0 mins /**Difficulty:** Easy

Serving Size: 0 servings

Ingredients:

- 1 lb. tuna steaks
- ¼ tsp. salt
- 2 tsp. olive oil
- 6 cups fresh baby spinach
- ¼ tsp. pepper
- ¾ cup frozen shelled edamame, thawed
- 1 cup grape tomatoes
- 2 tbsp. olive oil
- ½ cup frozen corn, thawed
- 1 tbsp. white wine vinegar
- 1 tbsp. minced fresh basil
- 1 tbsp. honey
- 1 tbsp. lemon juice
- 1 tbsp. lime juice
- 1 tbsp. orange juice
- 1/8 tsp. pepper
- 1/8 tsp. salt

Instructions:

Soak a kitchen towel with cooking oil and gently coat the grill rack with it, using long-handled tongs.

Season the tuna with salt and pepper after brushing it with olive oil. Cook for 2-3 minutes on each side, covered, over high temperature or broil 3-4 inches from the fire for rare; cook longer if preferred. Allow for a 5-minute rest period. Meanwhile, combine the tomatoes, spinach, edamame, and corn in a large mixing dish. Whisk together the olive oil, white wine vinegar, basil, lime juice, honey, lemon juice, and orange juice in a small bowl; sprinkle over salad and toss to cover. Salad should be divided among four dishes; tuna should be sliced and arranged over salads. Serve right away.

Nutritional Values: Calories: 294 kcal /Carbohydrates: 16 g /

Protein: 32 g /Fat: 12 g/Sodium: 306 mg

Lemon-Lime Salmon

Total Time: 20 mins / **Prep. Time:** 5 mins /**Cooking Time:** 1 mins /**Difficulty:** Easy

Serving Size: 6 servings

Ingredients:

- 6 salmon fillets
- ¼ tsp. salt
- ½ cup lime juice
- ½ cup lemon juice
- 1 tsp. seafood seasoning

Instructions:

In a 13x9-inch baking dish, place the salmon and add the lime and lemon juices. Season the salmon with salt and seafood seasoning. Bake it uncovered, at 425° for 10-15 minutes or until fish flakes readily with a fork.

Nutritional Values: Calories: 329 kcal /Carbohydrates: 25 g /

Protein: 27 g /Fat: 15 g/Sodium: 283mg

Shrimp Salad

Total Time: 15 mins / **Prep. Time:** 15 mins /**Cooking Time:** N/A /**Difficulty:** Easy

Serving Size: 4 servings

Ingredients:

- 5 oz. spring mix salad greens
- 1 large navel orange, sectioned

- 1 lb. cooked medium shrimp, deveined
- 1 cup fresh strawberries, quartered
- 1 medium ripe avocado, chopped
- Salad dressing of your choice
- ½ cup thinly sliced green onions

Instructions:

Arrange salad leaves, orange, shrimp, strawberries, avocado, and onions on each of four serving dishes. Dressing should be drizzled on top.

Nutritional Values: Calories: 239 kcal /Carbohydrates: 16 g /

Protein: 25 g /Fat: 9 g/Sodium: 181 mg

Savory Pork Salad

Total Time: 25 mins / **Prep. Time:** 15 mins /**Cooking Time:** 10 mins /**Difficulty:** Easy /**Serving Size:** 2 servings

Ingredients:

- 1 garlic clove, minced
- 2 tsp. olive oil
- ½ tsp. fresh gingerroot, minced
- 2 tsp. brown sugar
- ½ lb. pork tenderloin, thinly sliced
- 2 tsp. low-sodium soy sauce
- 2 tsp. minced fresh basil
- 1½ tsp. water
- 1½ tsp. lime juice
- 1 tsp. minced fresh oregano
- ½ cup grape tomatoes
- 3 cups torn mixed salad greens
- ½ small red onion, rings
- ½ yellow pepper, strips

Instructions:

Cook ginger and garlic in oil for 30 seconds in a large pan over medium heat. Cook and stir the pork until it is no longer pink. Remove from the oven and keep warm. Combine the basil, brown sugar, lime juice, soy sauce, water, and oregano in the same skillet. Bring the mixture to a boil. Turn off the heat. Combine the tomatoes, greens, yellow pepper, onion, and pork in a salad dish. Serve immediately after drizzling with warm dressing and tossing to coat.

Nutritional Values: Calories: 229 kcal /Carbohydrates: 13 g /

Protein: 25 g /Fat: 9 g/Sodium: 274 mg

Cobb Salad Wraps

Total Time: 15 mins / **Prep. Time:** 15 mins /**Cooking Time:** N/A /**Difficulty:** Easy

Serving Size: 4 servings

Ingredients:

- 2 cups cooked chicken breast, cubed
- 1 celery rib, thinly sliced
- ½ cup avocado, chopped
- 2 tbsp. chopped ripe olives
- ½ cup avocado, chopped
- 2 tbsp. lemon juice
- 2 tbsp. crumbled blue cheese
- 1½ tsp. Dijon mustard
- 1 tbsp. honey
- ¼ tsp. dill weed
- 1 garlic clove, minced
- 1/8 teaspoon pepper
- ¼ tsp. salt
- 1 tbsp. olive oil
- 4 whole wheat tortillas warmed
- 4 romaine leaves, torn
- 1 medium tomato, chopped

Instructions:

Combine the avocado, chicken, celery, olives, onion, and cheese in a small mixing bowl. Combine honey, lemon juice, mustard, dill weed, garlic, salt, and pepper in a separate small bowl. Oil should be whisked in. Toss the chicken mixture in the sauce to coat. Top each tortilla with romaine and 2/3 cup chicken mixture. Toss with tomato and wrap up.

Nutritional Values: Calories: 372 kcal /Carbohydrates: 32 g /

Protein: 29 g /Fat: 14 g/Sodium: 607 mg

Pork Grapefruit Stir-Fry

Total Time: 25 mins / **Prep. Time:** 15 mins /**Cooking Time:** 10 mins /**Difficulty:** Medium/**Serving Size:** 6 servings

Ingredients:

- 3 tbsp. cornstarch
- ¾ cup water
- ¾ cup grapefruit juice concentrate
- 1 tbsp. honey
- 3 tbsp. soy sauce
- 3 cups sliced zucchini
- ½ tsp. ground ginger

- 1 red or green pepper, julienned
- 1½ lb. pork tenderloin, strips
- 1 tbsp. canola oil
- 1 tbsp. sesame seeds, toasted
- 3 grapefruit, peeled and sectioned

Instructions:

Combine the grapefruit juice concentrate, cornstarch, soy sauce, water, honey, and ginger in a small dish and put aside. In a pan over medium-high heat, stir-fry red pepper and zucchini and in oil until crisp-tender. Remove from the oven and keep warm. Stir-fry until the pork is no longer pink, around 4 minutes. Remove from the oven and keep warm. Repeat with the rest of the pork. Bring the sauce to a boil in the skillet. Cook and stir for 2 minutes, or until the sauce has thickened. Return the pork and veggies to the pan and swirl to coat. In a small mixing bowl, gently fold in the grapefruit. Sesame seeds can be sprinkled on top.

Nutritional Values: Calories: 320 kcal /Carbohydrates: 39 g /

Protein: 27 g /Fat: 7 g/Sodium: 364 mg

Chicken Brunch Bake

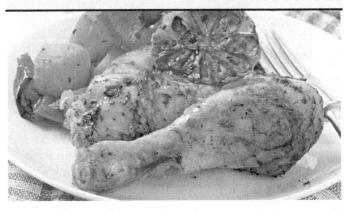

Total Time: 1 hour 15 mins / **Prep. Time:** 15 mins /**Cooking Time:** 1 hour /**Difficulty:** Medium/**Serving Size:** 8 servings

Ingredients:

- 3 cups chicken broth
- 9 slices day-old bread, cubed
- ½ cup uncooked instant rice
- 4 cups cooked chicken, cubed
- 2 tbsp. fresh parsley, minced
- ½ cup diced pimientos
- 4 large eggs, beaten
- ½ tsp. salt, optional

Instructions:

Toss bread cubes with broth in a large mixing dish. Combine the chicken, parsley, pimientos, rice, and salt, if preferred. Place the mixture in a greased 13x9-inch baking dish. Pour the eggs over everything. Preheat oven to 325°F and bake uncovered for 1 hour, or until a knife stuck in the middle comes out clean.

Nutritional Values: Calories: 233 kcal /Carbohydrates: 18 g /

Protein: 27 g /Fat: 6 g/Sodium: 458 mg

Cod with Hearty Tomato Sauce

Total Time: 30 mins / **Prep. Time:** 15 mins /**Cooking Time:** 15 mins /**Difficulty:** Medium/**Serving Size:** 4 servings

Ingredients:

- 2 cans diced tomatoes
- 2 tbsp. olive oil, divided
- 4 cod fillets
- ½ tsp. dried oregano
- 2 medium onions, thinly sliced
- ¼ tsp. crushed red pepper flakes
- ¼ tsp. pepper
- Minced fresh parsley, optional

Instructions:

In a blender, puree the tomatoes. Cover and purée them until smooth. Using paper towels, pat the fish dry. 1 tablespoon oil should be heated in a large pan over medium-high heat and add cod fillets in it. Cook until the surface of the cod fillets begins to brown, about 2-4 minutes each side. Remove the pan from the heat. Heat the remaining oil in the same skillet over medium-high heat. Cook and stir until onions are soft, about 2-4 minutes. Bring to a boil with the spices and pureed tomatoes. Return to a low boil and ladle sauce over tops of fish. Reduce heat to low and cook, uncovered, for 5-7 minutes, or until salmon flakes easily with a fork. Sprinkle with parsley if desired.

Nutritional Values: Calories: 271 kcal /Carbohydrates: 17 g /

Protein: 29 g /Fat: 8 g/Sodium: 784 mg

Spicy Coconut Shrimp with Quinoa

Total Time: 40 mins / **Prep. Time:** 20 mins /**Cooking Time:** 20 mins /**Difficulty:** Medium/**Serving Size:** 4 servings

Ingredients:

- 1 tsp. olive oil
- 1 cup quinoa, rinsed
- ¼ + ¼ tsp. salt
- 2 cups water
- 1 tbsp. minced fresh gingerroot
- 1 medium onion, chopped
- ½ tsp. ground cumin
- ½ tsp. curry powder
- ¼ tsp. cayenne pepper
- 2 cups fresh snow peas, trimmed
- 1 lb. uncooked shrimp
- 1 tbsp. orange juice
- ¼ cup minced fresh cilantro
- 3 tbsp. light coconut milk
- ¼ cup shredded coconut, toasted

Instructions:

Bring quinoa, water, and 1/4 tsp. salt to a boil in a large pot. Reduce heat to low; cover and cook for 12-15 minutes, or until liquid has been absorbed. Remove the pan from the heat and fluff with a fork. Meanwhile, heat the oil in a large nonstick pan over medium heat. Cook and stir for 4-6 minutes, or until onion is soft. Cook for a further minute after adding the curry powder, ginger, cumin, salt, and cayenne. In a large pan, sauté and toss the shrimp and snow peas for 3-4 minutes, or until the shrimp are pink and the snow peas are crisp-tender. Warm the coconut milk and orange juice. Serve with quinoa and a sprinkling of coconut and cilantro on top of each serving.

Nutritional Values: Calories: 330 kcal /Carbohydrates: 37 g /Protein: 26 g /Fat: 8 g/Sodium: 451 mg

Zippy Turkey Zoodles

Total Time: 45 mins / **Prep. Time:** 25 mins /**Cooking Time:** 20 mins /**Difficulty:** Medium/**Serving Size:** 4 servings

Ingredients:

- 4 tsp. olive oil, divided

- 1 small onion, finely chopped
- 1 lb. ground turkey
- 2 garlic cloves, minced
- 1 jalapeno pepper, chopped
- ½ tsp. salt
- ¾ tsp. ground cumin
- ¼ tsp. crushed red pepper flakes
- ¼ tsp. chili powder
- 4 plum tomatoes, chopped
- 3 medium zucchinis, spiralized
- ¼ tsp. pepper
- 1 cup black beans, rinsed and drained
- 1 cup frozen corn, thawed

Instructions:

2 tsp. olive oil should be heated in a large nonstick pan over medium heat Add the turkey, jalapeño, onion, and garlic and cook, breaking up the turkey into crumbles, until the turkey is no pinker and the veggies are cooked, about 8-10 minutes; drain. Season the mixture with salt and pepper, then remove from heat and keep warm. Wipe the pan clean. In the same pan, heat the remaining olive oil and sauté the zucchini until crisp-tender, about 3-5 minutes. Serve the corn, jalapeño, beans, and reserved turkey mixture with zucchini. If desired, garnish with cilantro and cheese.

Nutritional Values: Calories: 332 kcal /Carbohydrates: 26 g /

Protein: 29 g /Fat: 14 g/Sodium: 500 mg

Tuscan Fish Packets

Total Time: 30 mins / **Prep. Time:** 10 mins /**Cooking Time:** 20 mins /**Difficulty:** Medium/**Serving Size:** 4 servings

Ingredients:

- 15 oz. great northern beans, rinsed and drained
- 1 small zucchini, chopped
- 4 plum tomatoes, chopped
- 1 garlic clove, minced
- 1 medium onion, chopped
- ¾ tsp. salt, divided
- ¼ cup white wine
- 4 tilapia fillets
- ¼ tsp. pepper, divided
- 1 medium lemon, cut into 8 thin slices

Instructions:

Preheat the oven to 400°F. Combine the tomatoes, beans, onion, zucchini, garlic, wine, 1/2 tsp. salt, and 1/8 tsp. pepper in a large mixing dish. Clean the fish by rinsing it and patting it dry. Season each fillet with the remaining salt and pepper on an 18x12-inch sheet of heavy-duty foil. Serve the bean mixture over the fish with lemon slices on top. To seal the fish, fold the foil around it and crimp the edges. Place the packets on a baking sheet to cool. Bake for 15-20 minutes, or until the fish flakes easily with a fork and the veggies are soft. When opening packages, be cautious of leaking steam.

Nutritional Values: Calories: 270 kcal /Carbohydrates: 38 g /

Protein: 23 g /Fat: 2 g/Sodium: 653 mg

Italian Chicken

Total Time: 4 hour 20 mins / **Prep. Time:** 20 mins /**Cooking Time:** 4 hours /**Difficulty:** Medium/**Serving Size:** 4 servings

Ingredients:

- 4 skinless chicken breast halves
- 14 oz. stewed tomatoes, cut up
- 14 oz. low-sodium chicken broth
- 1 medium green pepper, chopped
- 8 oz. tomato sauce
- 1 garlic clove, minced
- 1 green onion, chopped
- 1 tsp. ground mustard
- 3 tsp. chili powder
- ¼ tsp. garlic powder
- ½ tsp. pepper
- 1/3 cup all-purpose flour
- ¼ tsp. onion powder
- ½ cup cold water

Instructions:

In a 3-quart slow cooker, place the chicken. Pour the broth, tomato sauce, tomatoes, onion, green pepper, garlic, and spices over the chicken. Cook on low for 4 hours or till meat is cooked, covered. Remove the chicken from the pan and keep it warm. Skim the fat from the cooking liquids and pour them into a large saucepan. Mix together the cold water and flour until smooth, then whisk in the juices. Bring to a boil, then reduce to a low heat and simmer, stirring constantly, for 2 minutes, or until the sauce has thickened.

Nutritional Values: Calories: 231 kcal /Carbohydrates: 22 g /

Protein: 28 g /Fat: 3 g/Sodium: 800 mg

Veggie And Hummus Sandwich

Total Time: 10 mins / **Prep. Time:** 10 mins /**Cooking Time:** N/A /**Difficulty:** Easy

Serving Size: 1 serving

Ingredients:

- 2 slices whole-grain bread
- ¼ avocado, mashed
- 3 tbsp. hummus
- ¼ medium red bell pepper, sliced
- ½ cup mixed salad greens
- ¼ cup shredded carrot
- ¼ cup sliced cucumber

Instructions:

Spread hummus on one slice of bread and avocado on the other. Greens, cucumber, bell pepper, and carrot should be added to the sandwich. Serve by slicing in half.

Nutritional Values: Calories: 325 kcal /Carbohydrates: 40 g /

Protein: 12 g /Fat: 14 g/Sodium: 407 mg

Salmon-Stuffed Avocados

Total Time: 15 mins / **Prep. Time:** 15 mins /**Cooking Time:** N/A /**Difficulty:** Easy

Serving Size: 4 servings

Ingredients:

- 2 avocados
- ½ cup nonfat plain Greek yogurt
- 2 tbsp. chopped fresh parsley
- 1 tbsp. lime juice
- ½ cup diced celery
- 1 tsp. Dijon mustard
- 2 tsp. mayonnaise
- 1/8 tsp. ground pepper
- 1/8 tsp. salt
- 10 oz. salmon, flaked
- Chopped chives for garnish

Instructions:

In a medium mixing bowl, combine the yoghurt, parsley, celery, lime juice, mustard, mayonnaise, salt, and pepper. Mix in the salmon well. Remove the pits from the avocados and cut them in half lengthwise. In a small dish, scoop roughly 1 tbsp. flesh from each avocado half. With a fork, mash the avocado flesh that has been scooped out and incorporate it into the salmon mixture. Fill each avocado half halfway with about 1/4 cup of the prepared salmon mixture, topdressing it on top. If desired, garnish with chives.

Nutritional Values: Calories: 293 kcal /Carbohydrates: 10 g /

Protein: 19 g /Fat: 22 g/Sodium: 400 mg

Egg Salad Sandwich

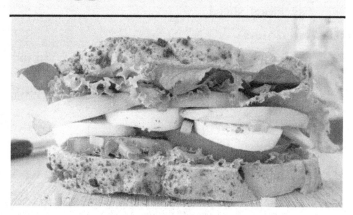

Total Time: 10 mins / **Prep. Time:** 5 mins /**Cooking Time:** 5 mins /**Difficulty:** Easy

Serving Size: 1 serving

Ingredients:

- 1 whole-wheat English muffin, split
- 2 medium carrots with tops
- 1 tsp. olive oil
- 1 tbsp. +1 tsp. mayonnaise
- 2 hard-boiled eggs
- 1 large romaine lettuce leaf, shredded

Instructions:

Preheat a nonstick grill pan or skillet over medium-high heat. Oil the cut edges of the English muffin halves. 1 to 2 minutes each side; grill the muffins till both sides are golden brown. Peel carrot and chop tops into sticks. Hard-boiled eggs should be diced and placed in a small bowl. Stir in the chopped carrot tops and mayonnaise until everything is well mixed. Fill the grilled muffin halves halfway with lettuce, then top with the egg salad. Carrots should be served on the side.

Nutritional Values: Calories: 497 kcal /Carbohydrates: 37 g /

Protein: 30 g /Fat: 20 g/Sodium: 548 mg

Catchall Lunch Salad

Total Time: 10 mins / **Prep. Time:** 10 mins /**Cooking Time:** N/A /**Difficulty:** Easy

Serving Size: 1 serving

Ingredients:

- 1½ cups sliced romaine
- 5 oz. can light tuna, drained
- ¾ cup rinsed canned chickpeas
- ½ cup cherry tomatoes, halved
- ½ cup coleslaw mix
- ¼ cup Easy Anchovy Vinaigrette
- 2 scallions, sliced

Instructions:

In a medium dish or food storage container, combine chickpeas, sliced romaine, tuna, coleslaw mix, tomatoes, and onions. Add the vinaigrette just before serving and toss to coat.

Nutritional Values: Calories: 488 kcal /Carbohydrates: 36 g /

Protein: 29 g /Fat: 24 g/Sodium: 650 mg

Quesadillas

Total Time: 20 mins / **Prep. Time:** 15 mins /**Cooking Time:** 5 mins /**Difficulty:** Medium/**Serving Size:** 4 servings

Ingredients:

- 2 oz. reduced-fat cream cheese, softened
- ½ avocado slices
- 4 whole wheat flour tortillas
- ½ tsp. adobo sauce
- ¼ cup green onions, chopped
- ½ cup red sweet pepper, chopped
- 4 tsp. jalapeño chile pepper, finely chopped
- cooking spray

Instructions:

Cream together adobo sauce and cream cheese in a small bowl until smooth. One half of each tortilla should be spread with the mixture. Sweet pepper, jalapeño chile pepper and green onions should be sprinkled over the cream cheese mixture. To make quesadillas, fold the unfilled side over. Spray a big nonstick skillet that hasn't been heated with nonstick cooking spray. Preheat the oven to 350°F. Cook quesadillas in batches of two for approximately 4 minutes, or until golden and cooked through, rotating halfway through. Cut in half crosswise. Avocado slices should be added on the top.

Nutritional Values: Calories: 132 kcal /Carbohydrates: 12 g /

Protein: 6 g /Fat: 7 g/Sodium: 265 mg

Egg And Broccoli Slaw Wrap

Total Time: 10 mins / **Prep. Time:** 10 mins /**Cooking Time:** N/A /**Difficulty:** Easy

Serving Size: 1 serving

Ingredients:

- 2 tbsp. light sour cream
- ¼ tsp. finely shredded lemon peel
- 1 tsp. chopped fresh chives
- ½ tsp. honey
- 1 tsp. lemon juice
- 2 hard-cooked eggs, sliced
- 1/3 cup shredded broccoli
- 2 tbsp. roasted red pepper, chopped
- 1 low-carb whole-wheat tortilla
- 1 dash ground pepper

Instructions:

In a small mixing dish, combine chives, sour cream, lemon juice, lemon peel, and honey. Toss in the broccoli slaw lightly to coat. Cover and chill for at least one night. Wrap egg slices in plastic wrap and refrigerate overnight. Leave a 1 1/2-inch gap on both ends of the broccoli mixture as you spread it over the bottom border of the tortilla. Serve with roasted pepper slices and egg pieces on top. If desired, season with freshly ground pepper. Fold the edges of the tortilla inwards over the contents. Begin rolling the tortilla from the bottom edge.

Nutritional Values: Calories: 272 kcal /Carbohydrates: 26 g /

Protein: 14 g /Fat: 21 g/Sodium: 438 mg

Mexican Roll-Ups

Total Time: 25 mins / **Prep. Time:** 10 mins /**Cooking Time:** 15 mins /**Difficulty:** Medium/**Serving Size:** 2 servings

Ingredients:

- 8 oz. extra-lean ground beef
- 1/3 cup chopped red sweet pepper
- 1/3 cup chopped tomato

- 1 tsp. ground cumin
- 1 tbsp. red wine vinegar
- 2 romaine lettuce leaves
- 1 tsp. olive oil
- 2 whole wheat tortillas

Instructions:

Cook ground beef in a medium pan over medium-high heat till cooked, breaking up the meat with a wooden spoon as it cooks. Remove any excess fat. In a pan, combine the sweet pepper, tomato, cumin, vinegar, and oil. On each tortilla, place a romaine leaf. On top of each lettuce leaf, spoon half of the prepared ground beef mixture. Roll up each filled tortilla completely. Using skewers fasten the roll-ups if desired.

Nutritional Values: Calories: 332 kcal /Carbohydrates: 28 g /

Protein: 29 g /Fat: 10 g/Sodium: 421 mg

Chapter 8: Dinner Recipes

People with diabetes of any sort do not have to give up their favorite meals in order to eat a healthy diet. The idea is to consume in moderation and maintain a healthy mix of proteins, carbs, and fats, with a focus on fiber.

Diabetes may be controlled with a mix of exercise, medical treatment, and proper food preparation. For persons with diabetes, dinner may be diverse, flavorful, and full. Dinner is an important part of our daily routine. The last meal of the day is critical for our physical well-being. It's also important in our social and familial lives. A decent dinner time may provide us with a healthy lifestyle as well as unforgettable times with our families.

In this chapter, we'll look at several delicious and healthy dinnertime choices for diabetics.

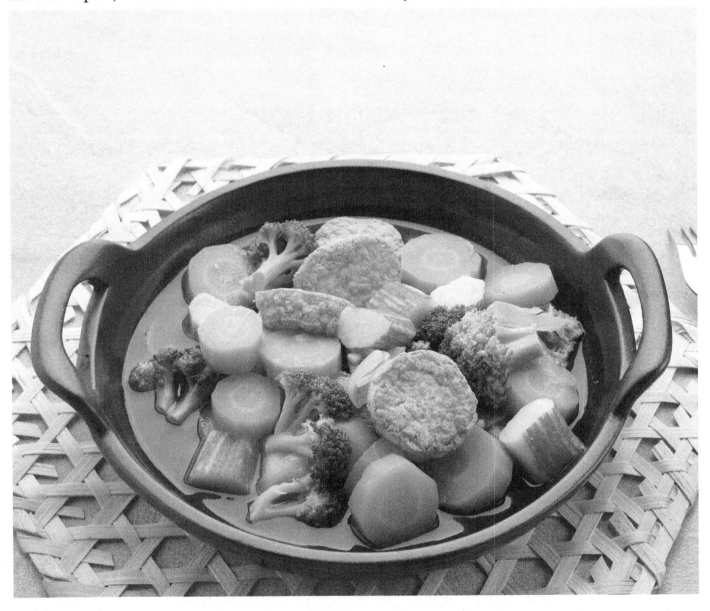

Stuffed Chicken Breast

Total Time: 25 mins / **Prep. Time:** 5 mins /**Cooking Time:** 20 mins /**Difficulty:** Medium/**Serving Size:** 1 serving

Ingredients:

- 1 chicken breast
- 1 artichoke heart
- 1 oz. low-fat mozzarella
- 5 large basil leaves
- 1 tsp. sundried tomato, chopped
- 1 clove garlic
- ¼ tsp. paprika
- pinch of pepper
- ¼ tsp. curry powder
- toothpicks

Instructions:

Preheat the oven to 365°F. Cut a slit lengthwise midway up the chicken breast to form a pocket for the stuffing. Cut the artichoke, mozzarella, tomato, basil, and garlic into small pieces. To combine, mix everything together. Stuff the prepared mixture into the pocket made in the chicken breast. Seal the chicken breast all around filling with toothpicks. Season the chicken breast with curry powder, pepper, and paprika and place it on a baking sheet or foil. Cook for around 20 minutes. Once done remove the toothpicks and serve!

Nutritional Values: Calories: 262 kcal /Carbohydrates: 8.5 g /

Protein: 46 g /Fat: 4 g/Sodium: 338 mg

Zucchini Lasagna

Total Time: 1 hour 30 mins / **Prep. Time:** 30 mins /**Cooking Time:** 1 hour /**Difficulty:** Hard/**Serving Size:** 4 servings

Ingredients:

- 16 oz. ground beef,
- 4½ oz. onion
- 2 medium zucchini
- 2 cloves garlic
- 3 tomatoes
- 1 serrano chili
- ½ cube Knorr chicken bouillon
- 5½ oz. mushrooms
- ½ cup low-fat mozzarella, shredded

- 1 tsp. dried thyme
- 1 tsp. dried basil
- Salt and pepper, to taste
- 1 tsp. paprika
- Cooking spray

Instructions:

Cut the zucchini into pieces with a julienne peeler. Leave aside for 10 minutes after lightly seasoning with salt. Use a paper towel to blot the zucchini slices. Grill or broil them for 3 minutes at high heat in the oven. Place the zucchini on paper towels after grilling or broiling. Make an X insertion in the top of the tomatoes by cutting off the ends. Place them in boiling water for several minutes, then drain and peel off the skin with cool water. Onions, chile, garlic, mushrooms and tomatoes should be roughly chopped. Coat a pan with cooking spray and sauté the onion, garlic, and chilli for 1 minute. In the same pan, add the mushrooms and tomatoes and cook for a further 4 minutes. Remove the vegetables from the heat and set them aside. In the same pan sauté the meat with the paprika until thoroughly cooked. Return the veggies to the pan, and then add the remaining spices and chicken bouillon. Allow the sauce to boil on low heat for 25 minutes. Preheat the oven to 375°F. Use 1/3 of the zucchini to form a layer in the bottom of a small baking pan lined with parchment paper. 1/3 of the meat sauce should go on top. Continue with another layer of zucchini until you've used up all of the sauce and zucchini. Bake for 35 minutes with shredded mozzarella on top. Remove the lasagna from the oven and set aside for 10 minutes to cool before serving.

Nutritional Values: Calories: 244 kcal /Carbohydrates: 12 g /

Protein: 30 g /Fat: 8 g/Sodium: 558 mg

Sweet and Tangy Salmon

Total Time: 35 mins / **Prep. Time:** 15 mins /**Cooking Time:** 20 mins /**Difficulty:** Easy /**Serving Size:** 4 servings

Ingredients:

- 4 salmon fillets
- 2 tbsp. brown sugar
- 1 tbsp. butter
- 2 tbsp. Dijon mustard
- 2 tbsp. low-sodium soy sauce
- ½ tsp. pepper
- 1/8 tsp. salt
- 1 tbsp. olive oil
- 1 lb. fresh green beans, trimmed

Instructions:

Preheat the oven to 425°F. Fill a 15x10-inch baking pan with fillets and spray with cooking spray. Melt butter in a small pan, and then add soy sauce, brown sugar, oil, mustard, pepper, and salt. Half of the sauce should be brushed over the fish. Toss green beans in a large mixing dish with the remaining brown sugar sauce to coat. Arrange green beans in a circle around the fillets. Roast for 14-16 minutes, or until green beans are crisp-tender and fish flakes easily with a fork.

Nutritional Values: Calories: 394 kcal /Carbohydrates: 17 g /

Protein: 31 g /Fat: 22 g/Sodium: 661 mg

Roasted Chicken and Vegetables

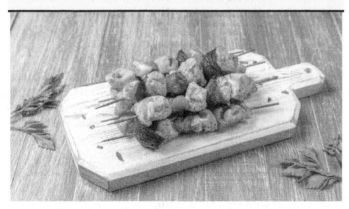

Total Time: 1 hour / **Prep. Time:** 15 mins /**Cooking Time:** 45 mins /**Difficulty:** Medium /**Serving Size:** 6 servings

Ingredients:

- 6 bone-in chicken thighs
- 6 medium red potatoes, cubed
- 2 tbsp. olive oil
- 1 large onion, chopped
- 1¼ tsp. salt, divided
- 3 garlic cloves, minced
- ¾ tsp. pepper, divided
- 1 tsp. dried rosemary, divided
- ½ tsp. paprika
- 6 cups baby spinach

Instructions:

Preheat the oven to 425°F. Toss onion, potatoes, oil, 3/4 tsp. salt, garlic, 1/2 tsp. rosemary, and 1/2 tsp. pepper in a large mixing bowl to coat. Place the coated vegetables in a baking pan that has been

sprayed with cooking spray. Combine paprika, the remaining rosemary, salt, and pepper in a small bowl. Toss the chicken with the paprika mixture and place it on top of the vegetables. Roast for 35-40 minutes, or until a thermometer placed in the chicken registers 170°-175° and the veggies are just tender. Transfer the chicken to a serving plate and set aside to keep warm. Add spinach to the veggies as a garnish. Roast for another 8-10 minutes, or until the veggies are soft and the spinach has wilted. Toss the vegetables together and serve with the chicken.

Nutritional Values: Calories: 357 kcal /Carbohydrates: 28 g /

Protein: 28 g /Fat: 14 g/Sodium: 597 mg

Peppered Tuna Kabobs

Total Time: 20 mins / **Prep. Time:** 10 mins /**Cooking Time:** 10 mins /**Difficulty:** Easy /**Serving Size:** 4 servings

Ingredients:

- 1 lb. tuna steaks, cubes
- 2 sweet red peppers, cubes
- 1 tsp. coarsely ground pepper
- 1 medium mango, cubes

Instructions:

Season the tuna with pepper. Thread mango tuna, and red peppers alternately on four metal or moistened wooden skewers. Skewers should be placed on a greased grill rack. Cook, over medium heat, stirring periodically, for 10 minutes, or until tuna is barely pink in the middle and peppers are soft.

Nutritional Values: Calories: 205 kcal /Carbohydrates: 20 g /

Protein: 29 g /Fat: 2 g/Sodium: 50 mg

Sesame Turkey Stir-Fry

Total Time: 25 mins / **Prep. Time:** 15 mins /**Cooking Time:** 10 mins /**Difficulty:** Easy /**Serving Size:** 4 servings

Ingredients:

- 1 tsp. cornstarch
- 2 tbsp. low-sodium soy sauce
- 2 tsp. curry powder
- ½ cup water
- 1/8 tsp. red pepper flakes
- 1 tbsp. honey

- 2 tsp. sesame oil
- 1 small onion, thinly sliced
- 1 sweet red pepper, julienned
- 1 green onion, sliced
- 2 cups cooked turkey breast, shredded
- 1 garlic clove, minced
- 2 cups cooked brown rice
- toasted sesame seeds, for garnish

Instructions:

Combine the first six ingredients in a small bowl until well combined. Heat the oil in a large skillet over medium-high heat. Stir in the onion and red pepper and until crisp-tender. Cook for a further minute after adding the garlic. Add the cornstarch mixture to the pan and stir well. Bring to a boil, then reduce to a low heat and simmer for 2 minutes, or until the sauce has thickened. Add the cooked turkey and give it a good mix. Add the green onion and mix well. Serve with a side of rice. Top with sesame seeds and enjoy.

Nutritional Values: Calories: 269 kcal /Carbohydrates: 32 g /

Protein: 25 g /Fat: 4 g/Sodium: 349 mg

Curry Turkey Stir-Fry

Total Time: 20 mins / **Prep. Time:** 10 mins /**Cooking Time:** 10 mins /**Difficulty:** Easy /**Serving Size:** 4 servings

Ingredients:

- ½ tsp. cornstarch
- 1 tbsp. fresh cilantro, minced
- 2 tbsp. low-sodium soy sauce
- 1 tsp. curry powder
- 1 garlic clove, minced
- 1 tbsp. honey
- 1 tsp. sesame oil
- 1/8 tsp. crushed red pepper flakes
- 1 sweet red pepper, julienned
- 3 green onions
- 2 cups cooked turkey breast, cubed
- 1 tbsp. canola oil
- 2 cups cooked brown rice

Instructions:

Combine the first eight ingredients and make a sauce. Heat canola oil in a large pan over medium-high heat and stir-fry red pepper for 2 minutes, until crisp-tender. Stir in green onions and cook for 1-2 minutes, or until tender. Add the cornstarch sauce to the pan and stir well. Bring to a boil, then simmer and stir for 1-2 minutes, or until the sauce has thickened. Heat

thoroughly the turkey by stirring it in. Serve with a side of rice.

Nutritional Values: Calories: 287 kcal /Carbohydrates: 31 g /

Protein: 25 g /Fat: 7 g/Sodium: 351 mg

Cajun Beef and Rice

Total Time: 35 mins / **Prep. Time:** 10 mins /**Cooking Time:** 25 mins /**Difficulty:** Medium /**Serving Size:** 4 servings

Ingredients:

- 1 lb. lean ground beef
- 1 green pepper, chopped
- 3 celery ribs, chopped
- ¼ cup chopped onion
- 1 sweet red pepper, chopped
- 1 cup instant brown rice
- 2 cups water
- 1 tbsp. Worcestershire sauce
- 1 tbsp. fresh parsley, minced
- 1 tsp. Cajun seasoning
- 2 tsp. low-sodium beef bouillon
- ¼ tsp. crushed red pepper flakes
- 1/8 tsp. garlic powder
- ¼ tsp. black pepper

Instructions:

Cook celery, beef, onion, green and red peppers, in a large pan over medium heat for 10 minutes until beef is no longer pink; crumble the beef; drain. Combine the remaining ingredients in the pan. Bring to the boil. Reduce heat to low and cook, covered, for 12-15 minutes, or until rice is tender.

Nutritional Values: Calories: 291 kcal /Carbohydrates: 23 g /

Protein: 25 g /Fat: 10 g/Sodium: 422 mg

Cheesy Crispy Diabetic Pizza

Total Time: 14 mins / **Prep. Time:** 10 mins /**Cooking Time:** 4 mins /**Difficulty:** Easy /**Serving Size:** 1 serving

Ingredients:

- 1 tsp. olive oil
- 5 pepperonis
- 3 tbsp. pizza sauce

- 1 tortilla, low carb
- 1/3 cup cheese
- ¼ tsp. oregano leaves, optional

Instructions:

Preheat the oven to broil. In a big iron skillet, heat the olive oil. Heat the tortilla in a pan for 2-3 minutes, or until it is browned and crispy. After flipping the tortilla to the opposite side, add the sauce and pepperoni. If desired, sprinkle with oregano leaves. Place pan in oven for a few minutes, or until cheese melts and the sides of the tortillas begin to brown. Depending on your oven, it will take about 2-3 minutes. To avoid overcooking, keep a constant eye on the pizza. Slice the pizza after transferring it to the serving pan.

Nutritional Values: Calories: 313 kcal /Carbohydrates: 15 g /

Protein: 14 g /Fat: 21 g/Sodium: 764 mg

Beef and Veggie Chili

Total Time: 50 mins / **Prep. Time:** 10 mins /**Cooking Time:** 40 mins /**Difficulty:** Medium/**Serving Size:** 6 servings

Ingredients:

- ½ lb. lean ground beef
- 1 tsp. olive oil
- 1 clove garlic, minced
- 1 small onion, chopped
- 2 stalks celery, chopped
- 1 carrot, chopped
- ½ tsp. salt
- 1 small bell pepper, chopped
- ½ tbsp. chili powder
- ½ tbsp. cumin
- 15 oz. can kidney beans, rinsed
- ¼ tsp. cinnamon
- 2/3 cup chicken broth, low- sodium
- 14.5 oz. can diced tomatoes, with liquid
- ¾ cup mild rotel
- sour cream, optional
- salt and pepper to taste
- grated cheese, optional

Instructions:

In a medium soup pot, heat the oil, and then add the onion, beef, garlic, celery, carrot, and bell pepper. Over medium heat, cook and stir until the meat is browned. Stir with the remaining ingredients. Seasonings can be adjusted as needed. Simmer for 30 minutes on low heat. If desired, top with shredded

cheese and sour cream.

Nutritional Values: Calories: 113 kcal /Carbohydrates: 20 g /Protein: 13 g /Fat: 5 g/Sodium: 534 mg

Chicken Ricotta

Total Time: 30 mins / **Prep. Time:** 15 mins /**Cooking Time:** 15 mins /**Difficulty:** Medium /**Serving Size:** 4 servings

Ingredients:

- 1 lb. chicken tenders
- 1 tbsp. olive oil
- ½ cup parmesan cheese
- 1 cup ricotta cheese
- 1 cup cherry tomatoes, roasted
- 1 tsp. oregano, crushed
- Spiralized yellow squash, lightly sautéed
- olives, garnish optional

Instructions:

Sauté chicken tenders with olive oil in a skillet. Parmesan, Ricotta, and oregano are combined in a small bowl. To blend, stir everything together. Spirals of yellow squash should be combined with olive oil and season with salt and pepper to taste. To assemble, spread ricotta cheese mixture over chicken tenders and top with roasted tomatoes. To heat, place under the broiler. Serve with Squash mixture.

Nutritional Values: Calories: 271 kcal /Carbohydrates: 5 g /

Protein: 36 g /Fat: 11 g/Sodium: 589 mg

Greek Yogurt Chicken

Total Time: 2 hours / **Prep. Time:** 1 hour /**Cooking Time:** 1 hour /**Difficulty:** Medium /**Serving Size:** 5 servings

Ingredients:

- 2 lb. chicken pieces
- 1 tbsp. olive oil
- ½ cup plain Greek yogurt
- ½ tsp. minced garlic
- ½ tbsp. lemon juice
- ¼ tsp. cinnamon
- ½ tsp. curry powder
- Pinch of salt and pepper
- 3 tbsp. Butter

Instructions:

Place the chicken in a big plastic bag with a zipper. Combine yogurt, lemon juice, oil, curry powder, garlic, salt, cinnamon, and pepper in a small bowl. Place the ingredients in a plastic bag with the chicken and marinate for at least 1 hour. Preheat the oven to 375°F. Heat 3 tsp. butter in a medium iron or oven-proof skillet over medium heat until butter melts. Brown a couple pieces of chicken in a skillet for about 4-5 minutes each side. As the chicken browns, remove it to a dish and add more pieces to the skillet until all of the chicken is browned. Return all chicken pieces to the skillet and roast for 40-50 minutes, or until thoroughly done.

Nutritional Values: Calories: 237 kcal /Carbohydrates: 1 g /

Protein: 19 g /Fat: 16 g/Sodium: 72 mg

Mediterranean Chicken

Total Time: 35 mins / **Prep. Time:** 10 mins /**Cooking Time:** 25 mins /**Difficulty:** Medium /**Serving Size:** 4 servings

Ingredients:

- 2 tsp. olive oil, divided
- salt and pepper, to taste
- 1 tsp. crushed oregano
- ¼ cup chopped onions
- 4 chicken thighs
- 6 small mushrooms sliced
- 2 garlic cloves minced
- 1/3 cup feta cheese
- 1 cup fresh spinach, chopped
- ¼ cup sun dried tomatoes, sliced
- 1/3 cup Italian cheese, grated

Instructions:

In an oven-safe skillet, heat 1 tsp. olive oil. Season the chicken thighs with pepper, salt, and oregano. Then brown on each side in a hot skillet. Remove the pan from the heat. Cook the garlic, onions and mushrooms until tender in another tsp. of olive oil in the skillet. Sun-dried tomatoes, spinach, feta, and browned chicken are then added to the vegetables mix. Italian cheese should be sprinkled on top. Preheat oven to 350°F and bake skillet for 20-30 minutes, or until done. At 165°F, the chicken is thoroughly cooked. Allow 5 minutes for flavors to meld before serving.

Nutritional Values: Calories: 362 kcal /Carbohydrates: 8 g /

Protein: 25 g /Fat: 26 g/Sodium: 269 mg

Chicken Alfredo

Total Time: 20 mins / **Prep. Time:** 5 mins /**Cooking Time:** 15 mins /**Difficulty:** Easy /**Serving Size:** 2 servings

Ingredients:

- 1 tsp. olive oil
- 1 tsp. minced garlic
- 1 green onion
- 1 cup portabella mushrooms, sliced
- 2 cups chopped fresh spinach
- 1 cup diced cherry tomatoes
- 5 grilled chicken tenders, chopped
- 2 summer squash, spiralized
- 1/3 cup alfredo sauce

Instructions:

In a large nonstick skillet, heat the oil. Add the garlic, green onion, and mushrooms in the skillet. Cook the vegetables for 3–4 minutes, or until the mushrooms are soft. Sauté the tomatoes and spinach until the spinach wilts little. Stir in the chicken. Stir Alfredo sauce into everything. Serve with spiralized squash.

Nutritional Values: Calories: 270 kcal /Carbohydrates: 7 g /

Protein: 30 g /Fat: 12 g/Sodium: 455 mg

Cabbage and Meat Gravy

Total Time: 30 mins / **Prep. Time:** 10 mins /**Cooking Time:** 20 mins /**Difficulty:** Easy /**Serving Size:** 4 servings

Ingredients:

- 1 tsp. olive oil
- 1 clove garlic, minced
- 1 small onion, chopped
- 3 cups chopped cabbage
- 14.5 oz. can diced tomatoes
- 1 lb. lean ground beef
- ¼ tsp. cinnamon
- 8 oz. low carb marinara
- ¼ tsp. salt

Instructions:

Heat the oil in a big pan, then add the onions and cook for 2-3 minutes. Garlic and ground meat should be added at this point. Brown the ground beef in a skillet, then drain the fat before adding the tomatoes, marinara, and spices. Stir in the cabbage until everything is well combined. Bring to a low boil, and then reduce to a low heat and cover. Cook it for 15-20 minutes, or until the cabbage is tender. Serve without rice for a low-carb supper, or with rice for a family-friendly meal.

Nutritional Values: Calories: 280 kcal /Carbohydrates: 16 g /Protein: 26 g /Fat: 12 g/Sodium: 663 mg

Italian Beef and Cheese Bowl

Total Time: 30 mins / **Prep. Time:** 15 mins /**Cooking Time:** 15 mins /**Difficulty:** Medium /**Serving Size:** 5 servings

Ingredients:

- 4 tsp. olive oil, divided
- 4 green onions, chopped
- ½ tsp. minced garlic
- 1½ lb. steak
- ½ cup pepperoncini, chopped
- 4 slices provolone cheese
- 2 tsp. Worcestershire sauce
- romaine lettuce leaves, for serving
- sliced tomatoes, for serving

Instructions:

In a pan, heat 2 tsp. olive oil until hot, and then add the onions, garlic, and pepperoncini peppers. Cook for 4-5 minutes, stirring periodically, until the vegetables are soft. Remove the pan from the heat and set it aside. Cut the steak into strips and mix in Worcestershire sauce. In a pan, heat the remaining olive oil, and then add the steak strips in stages. Brown each side of the steak before removing it from the skillet. Toss the meat and pepperoncini mixture back into the skillet to incorporate. Place four pieces of provolone cheese on top of everything. Allow the cheese to melt in the covered pan. Serve with sliced tomatoes, romaine lettuce leaves, and other garnishes.

Nutritional Values: Calories: 373 kcal /Carbohydrates: 2 g /Protein: 32 g /Fat: 27 g/Sodium: 231 mg

Pork Chops with Mexican Rice

Total Time: 30 mins / **Prep. Time:** 10 mins /**Cooking Time:** 20 mins /**Difficulty:** Easy

/**Serving Size:** 6 servings

Ingredients:

- 1 lb. boneless pork chops
- salt and pepper, to taste
- 1½ tbsp. olive oil, divided
- 2 green onions, diced
- 1 cup peppers, diced
- 1¼ cup chicken broth
- 1 cup rice
- ¾ cup salsa
- ½ cup cheddar cheese

Instructions:

Heat 1 tbsp. olive oil in a large pan over medium heat. Season the pork chops with salt and pepper to taste. Brown pork chops in hot oil for 1-2 minutes per side, then put aside. Over medium heat, add the remaining 1/2 tbsp. oil to the skillet and sauté the peppers and onions for 1-2 minutes. Continue to sauté until the rice is slightly browned. Stir with the remaining ingredients. Arrange pork chops on top of rice in pan and cover. Bring the rice and pork chops to a low simmer and cook for 15-20 minutes, or until the rice is done and the pork chops are thoroughly cooked. Top with cheese and let aside to melt.

Nutritional Values: Calories: 323 kcal /Carbohydrates: 28 g /Protein: 23 g /Fat: 13 g/Sodium: 535 mg

Quick and Easy Vegetable Curry

Total Time: 45 mins / **Prep. Time:** 10 mins /**Cooking Time:** 35 mins /**Difficulty:** Medium/**Serving Size:** 4 servings

Ingredients:

- 1 tbsp. olive oil
- 2 cloves crushed garlic
- 1 onion, chopped
- 2 tbsp. tomato paste
- 2 tbsp. chopped fresh cilantro
- 2½ tbsp. curry powder
- 1 cube vegetable bouillon
- 14 oz. can tomato, diced
- 1½ cups water
- 10 oz. frozen mixed vegetables
- salt and pepper to taste

Instructions:

Heat the oil in a big saucepan over medium-high heat

and cook the onion and garlic until golden. Cook for 2 to 3 minutes after adding the tomato paste and curry powder. Toss in the vegetable bouillon cube, tomatoes, mixed veggies, water, and season to taste with salt and pepper. Cook for 30 minutes, or until veggies are tender (not crunchy). Before serving, garnish with fresh cilantro.

Nutritional Values: Calories: 103 kcal /Carbohydrates: 15 g /Protein: 3 g /Fat: 3 g/Sodium: 266 mg

Hawaiian Chicken Packets

Total Time: 50 mins / **Prep. Time:** 20 mins /**Cooking Time:** 30 mins /**Difficulty:** Easy /**Serving Size:** 4 servings

Ingredients:

- 4 skinless, chicken breast halves
- 1 green bell pepper, sliced
- 1 cup teriyaki sauce
- 1 onion, chopped
- 1 red bell pepper, sliced
- 20 oz. can pineapple chunks, drained

Instructions:

Preheat the grill to medium-high. Place four squares of aluminum foil on the counter. In the center of each square, place one piece of chicken. Turn them over in the teriyaki sauce to coat them. Distribute the red and green peppers, onion, and pineapple slices among the chicken pieces in equal numbers. Fold the foil in half and tuck it inside the packages. Cook for about 20 minutes on the grill, or until the chicken is no longer pink and the juices flow clear.

Nutritional Values: Calories: 304 kcal /Carbohydrates: 38 g /Protein: 33 g /Fat: 1 g/Sodium: 284 mg

Spicy Chicken Breasts

Total Time: 30 mins / **Prep. Time:** 15 mins /**Cooking Time:** 15 mins /**Difficulty:** Easy /**Serving Size:** 4 servings

Ingredients:

- 2½ tbsp. paprika
- 1 tbsp. salt
- 2 tbsp. garlic powder
- 1 tbsp. dried thyme

- 1 tbsp. onion powder
- 1 tbsp. ground black pepper
- 1 tbsp. ground cayenne pepper
- 4 skinless, chicken breast halves

Instructions:

Combine the garlic powder, paprika, onion powder, salt, cayenne pepper, thyme, and ground black pepper in a medium mixing bowl. 3 tbsp. of the spice combination should be set aside for the chicken; the rest should be stored in an airtight container for later use. Preheat the grill to medium-high. On both sides of the chicken breasts, rub the spice mixture. Grease the grill grate lightly. Grill the chicken for 6 to 8 minutes per side, or until the juices run clear.

Nutritional Values: Calories: 173 kcal /Carbohydrates: 9 g /Protein: 29 g /Fat: 2 g/Sodium: 184 mg

Cinnamon Chicken

Total Time: 40 mins / **Prep. Time:** 10 mins /**Cooking Time:** 30 mins /**Difficulty:** Easy /**Serving Size:** 4 servings

Ingredients:

- 4 skinless, chicken breast halves
- 2 tbsp. Italian-style seasoning
- 1 tsp. ground cinnamon
- 3 tsp. salt
- 1½ tsp. garlic powder
- 1 tsp. ground black pepper

Instructions:

Preheat the oven to 350°F. Place the chicken in a 9x13 inch baking dish that has been lightly oiled. Season with seasoning, ground cinnamon, salt, garlic powder, and pepper, and mix well. Bake for 30 minutes at 350°F or until chicken is baked through and juices flow clear.

Nutritional Values: Calories: 143 kcal /Carbohydrates: 3 g /Protein: 27 g /Fat: 1 g/Sodium: 188 mg

Chicken Tenders

Total Time: 15 mins / **Prep. Time:** 5 mins /**Cooking Time:** 10 mins /**Difficulty:** Easy /**Serving Size:** 4 servings

Ingredients:

- 1 lb. chicken tenders
- seasoning salt, to taste

- 2 tsp. olive oil

Instructions:

Preheat your air fryer to 380°F. Season the chicken tenders generously with seasoning salt after tossing them in oil. Bake for 8-10 minutes. Serve and enjoy.

Nutritional Values: Calories: 147 kcal /Carbohydrates: 0 g /Protein: 24 g /Fat: 5 g/Sodium: 132 mg

Chicken Wings

Total Time: 35 mins / **Prep. Time:** 5 mins /**Cooking Time:** 30 mins /**Difficulty:** Easy /**Serving Size:** 4 servings

Ingredients:

- 2 lb. Chicken wings
- Salt, to taste

Instructions:

Preheat your air fryer for 5 minutes at 350°F. Dry out the moisture out from chicken wings and season with salt. Cook for 12 minutes in the air fryer, aiming to leave some gap between each chicken wing. Cook for another 12 minutes on the opposite side. Raise the temperature to 400°F and continue to cook for another 3-5 minutes, or until crisp and brown.

Nutritional Values: Calories: 440 kcal /Carbohydrates: 5 g /Protein: 34 g /Fat: 34 g/Sodium: 400 mg

Basil-Lime Scallops

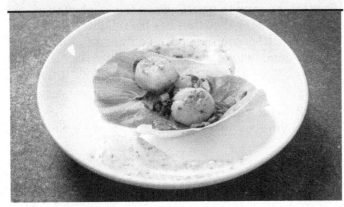

Total Time: 20 mins / **Prep. Time:** 15 mins /**Cooking Time:** 5 mins /**Difficulty:** Easy /**Serving Size:** 4 servings

Ingredients:

- 2 tbsp. chopped fresh basil
- 1 tsp. low-sodium soy sauce

- 1 lime juice
- 1 clove garlic, minced
- 1 tsp. vegetable oil
- 8 jumbo sea scallops
- 1/8 tsp. red pepper flakes
- Mixed baby greens, for garnish
- Lime wedges, for garnish

Instructions:

In a shallow bowl, whisk lime juice, basil, oil, soy sauce, garlic, and red pepper flakes until smooth and thoroughly combined. Add the scallops and flip them to evenly coat them. Over medium-high heat, heat a large nonstick skillet. Cook scallops for 3 minutes each side, or until done to your liking. On each serving plate, arrange 2 scallops. Serve with mixed greens and lime wedges as a garnish.

Nutritional Values: Calories: 92 kcal /Carbohydrates: 5 g /Protein: 14 g /Fat: 2 g/Sodium: 495 mg

Shrimp and Pineapple Kabobs

Total Time: 15 mins / **Prep. Time:** 10 mins /**Cooking Time:** 5 mins /**Difficulty:** Easy /**Serving Size:** 4 servings

Ingredients:

- ½ lb. medium raw shrimp, peeled and deveined
- ¼ tsp. garlic powder
- ½ cup pineapple juice
- 1 green bell pepper, 1-inch pieces
- 12 chunks canned pineapple
- ¼ cup prepared chili sauce

Instructions:

In a medium mixing dish, combine the shrimp, lemon juice, and garlic powder; toss to coat. Drain the shrimp and toss out the marinade. Thread pepper, pineapple, and shrimp alternately onto 4 (10-inch) skewers. Chili sauce should be brushed on. Grill for 5 minutes, or until shrimp are opaque, 4 inches from fire, flipping once and basting with chili sauce.

Nutritional Values: Calories: 100 kcal /Carbohydrates: 14 g /Protein: 10 g /Fat: 1 g/Sodium: 302 mg

Fresh Garlic Shrimp Linguine

Total Time: 20 mins / **Prep. Time:** 10 mins /**Cooking Time:** 10 mins /**Difficulty:** Medium/**Serving Size:** 4 servings

Ingredients:

- 6 oz. multigrain linguine, uncooked
- ¼ cup grated Parmesan cheese
- ½ lb. raw shrimp, peeled and deveined
- 1 clove garlic, minced
- 3 tbsp. diet margarine
- ¼ cup fresh parsley, chopped
- ½ tsp. seafood seasoning
- 1/8 tsp. salt

Instructions:

Cook linguine as directed on the box, eliminating salt and fat, for about 7 minutes or till al dente. Add the shrimp and simmer for 3 to 4 minutes, or until pink and opaque. Drain and place in a medium mixing bowl. Toss lightly to mix with margarine, cheese, garlic, and seafood flavor seasoning. Toss in the parsley and serve.

Nutritional Values: Calories: 270 kcal /Carbohydrates: 30 g /

Protein: 21 g /Fat: 7 g/Sodium: 242 mg

Sautéed Shrimp

Total Time: 15 mins / **Prep. Time:** 10 mins /**Cooking Time:** 5 mins /**Difficulty:** Easy /**Serving Size:** 2 servings

Ingredients:

- 4 sun-dried tomato halves
- 1 tbsp. olive oil
- ¼ cup hot water
- 1 cup baby spinach leaves
- ½ lb. cooked and peeled shrimp
- ¼ tsp. black pepper
- 1 tsp. dried basil

Instructions:

In a small dish, combine the sun-dried tomato halves. Set aside for 10 minutes, turning regularly, after pouring boiling water over the tomatoes. Remove the tomatoes from the water after 10 minutes, keeping the water for later use. Set aside chopped tomatoes. Heat olive oil in a big sauté pan and sauté the cooked shrimp. Cook for a few minutes after adding the spinach and chopped tomato, then add the 1/4 cup of boiling water that was set aside. Stir in the black pepper and dried basil until well blended, then serve right away.

Nutritional Values: Calories: 180 kcal /Carbohydrates: 4 g /Protein: 25 g /Fat: 8 g/Sodium: 346 mg

Grilled Rosemary Chicken

Total Time: 20 mins / **Prep. Time:** 10 mins /**Cooking Time:** 10 mins /**Difficulty:** Easy /**Serving Size:** 4 servings

Ingredients:

- 4 skinless chicken breasts
- Nonstick cooking spray
- 2 tbsp. lemon juice
- 2 tbsp. minced fresh rosemary leaves
- 2 cloves garlic, minced
- 2 tbsp. olive oil
- ¼ tsp. salt

Instructions:

Spray nonstick cooking spray on the chilly grill grid. Make sure the grill is ready for direct grilling. In a small bowl, combine lemon juice, rosemary, oil, garlic, and salt. Pour the mixture into a shallow glass dish. Turn the chicken to cover both sides with the lemon juice mixture. Cover and marinate for 15 minutes in the refrigerator, flipping chicken once. Remove the chicken and toss out the marinade. 5 to 6 minutes per side over medium-hot coals, or until chicken is no more pinkish in the center. If preferred, serve with grilled or steaming fresh veggies.

Nutritional Values: Calories: 192 kcal /Carbohydrates: 2 g /

Protein: 26 g /Fat: 8 g/Sodium: 222 mg

Orange-Glazed Pork Chops

Total Time: 30 mins / **Prep. Time:** 10 mins /**Cooking Time:** 20 mins /**Difficulty:** Medium/**Serving Size:** 4 servings

Ingredients:

- 2 tsp. olive oil
- ¼ cup orange juice
- 3 cups butternut squash, cubed

- ¼ cup dried cranberries
- 4 tbsp. low-sugar orange marmalade, divided
- ¼ tsp. salt
- 4 boneless center-cut pork chops
- ¼ tsp. black pepper

Instructions:

In a large nonstick skillet, heat the oil over medium heat. Cook, covered, for 15 minutes or until squash is soft, stirring occasionally. Combine the 2-tbsp. orange marmalade, orange juice, and the cranberries in a mixing bowl. Cook it for 1 minute, uncovered, or until almost all of the liquid has evaporated. Heat a big heavy pan over medium heat in the meantime. Season pork chops with salt and pepper, then cook for 3 to 4 minutes per side, or until the center is slightly pink. Add the remaining 2 tbsp. marmalade and flip the chops until evenly covered as the marmalade melts. Serve the pork with a side of squash.

Nutritional Values: Calories: 265 kcal /Carbohydrates: 23 g /Protein: 26 g /Fat: 8 g/Sodium: 209 mg

Grilled Chicken Adobo

Total Time: 55 mins / **Prep. Time:** 30 mins /**Cooking Time:** 15 mins /**Difficulty:** Medium/**Serving Size:** 6 servings

Ingredients:

- ½ cup chopped onion
- 6 cloves garlic, coarsely chopped
- 1/3 cup lime juice
- 1 tsp. dried oregano
- 1 tsp. ground cumin
- ¼ tsp. ground red pepper
- ½ tsp. dried thyme
- 3 tbsp. chopped fresh cilantro, for garnish
- 6 skinless chicken breasts

Instructions:

In a food processor, combine the lime juice, onion and garlic. Using a food processor, finely chop the onion. Fill a big resealable food storage bag halfway with the mixture. Mix in the oregano, cumin, red pepper and thyme until well combined. Place the chicken in the bag, squeeze out the air, and close it. Turn the chicken to coat it with the marinade. Refrigerate for 30 minutes, rotating once or twice. Using nonstick frying spray, coat the grid. Make sure the grill is ready for direct grilling. Remove the chicken from the marinade and discard it. Arrange the chicken on the grid. Over medium heat, grill 5 to 7 minutes on each side, or until chicken is no more pinkish in the center. Transfer to a clean serving tray and garnish with cilantro.

Nutritional Values: Calories: 139 kcal /Carbohydrates: 1 g /Protein: 25 g /Fat: 3 g/Sodium: 61 mg

Orange Chicken

Total Time: 20 mins / **Prep. Time:** 10 mins /**Cooking Time:** 10 mins /**Difficulty:** Medium/**Serving Size:** 4 servings

Ingredients:

- 2 tbsp. frozen orange juice concentrate
- 1 tsp. Dijon mustard
- 1 tbsp. orange marmalade, no-sugar-added
- 4 skinless chicken breast halves
- ¼ tsp. salt
- 2 tbsp. chopped fresh parsley
- ½ cup fresh orange sections

Instructions:

In an 8-inch shallow microwavable dish, mix the juice concentrate, mustard, marmalade, and salt until the juice concentrate has thawed. Add the chicken and cover it in the sauce on both sides. Arrange chicken around the dish's edge, not overlapping it. Cover with plastic wrap that has been ventilated. Microwave on high for 3 minutes, and then flip the chicken. Microwave on high for 4 minutes or until chicken is no more pinkish in the center. Place the chicken on a serving platter. Microwave the sauce for 2 to 3 minutes on high, or until slightly thickened. Pour sauce over chicken and garnish with orange pieces and parsley.

Nutritional Values: Calories: 157 kcal /Carbohydrates: 8 g /

Protein: 27 g /Fat: 1 g/Sodium: 234 mg

Lemon Caper Tilapia

Total Time: 14 mins / **Prep. Time:** 5 mins /**Cooking Time:** 9 mins /**Difficulty:** Easy

Serving Size: 2 servings

Ingredients:

- Cooking spray
- 2 tilapia fillets
- 2 tsp. reduced-fat margarine
- ½ tsp. lemon zest
- 1 tsp. fresh-squeezed lemon juice

- 1 tbsp. capers
- 1 tbsp. white wine

Instructions:

Warm a nonstick skillet over medium heat with cooking spray. In a pan, melt the margarine, and then add the tilapia fillets. Cook for 2–3 mins on each side, or until a fork pierced the fish readily flakes. Cover and keep the fish warm in a serving dish. Add the lemon zest, lemon juice, wine, and capers to the skillet and mix to blend. Cook for 1 minute before pouring over the fish.

Nutritional Values: Calories: 115 kcal /Carbohydrates: 1 g /

Protein: 21 g /Fat: 3 g/Sodium: 220 mg

Basil Grilled Shrimp

Total Time: 36 mins / **Prep. Time:** 30 mins /**Cooking Time:** 6 mins /**Difficulty:** Medium/**Serving Size:** 6 servings

Ingredients:

- 1 tbsp. olive oil
- 1 lb. medium fresh shrimp
- ½ lemon juice
- 1 tbsp. coarse-grain prepared mustard
- 1½ tbsp. reduced-calorie margarine, melted
- 1 clove garlic, minced
- 1 cup fresh basil, minced
- pinch of black pepper
- Cooking spray

Instructions:

Whisk together margarine, olive oil, mustard, lemon juice, garlic, basil, and pepper in a small bowl; transfer to a large zip-top bag. Toss in the shrimp and gently toss to coat. Refrigerate for 1 hour to marinate. Heat the grill to medium-high. Remove the shrimp from the sauce and skewer them. Spray the grill grate with nonstick cooking spray. Place the skewers on the grill over medium high heat and sprinkle with any leftover marinade. Cook for 2–3 minutes, then flip the shrimp and cook for another 2–3 minutes, or until pink and opaque.

Nutritional Values: Calories: 180 kcal /Carbohydrates: 3 g /Protein: 24 g /Fat: 8 g/Sodium: 280 mg

Herb Marinated Chicken

Total Time: 50 mins / **Prep. Time:** 30 mins

/**Cooking Time:** 20 mins /**Difficulty:** Medium/**Serving Size:** 6 servings

Ingredients:

- 1½ lb. boneless, skinless chicken breasts
- ½ cup balsamic vinegar
- ¼ cup olive oil
- ½ tsp. dry parsley
- 3 cloves garlic, minced
- ¾ tsp. dry sage
- 1 tsp. dry rosemary
- 1 tsp. salt
- 1 tsp. dry thyme
- ½ tsp. coarse ground pepper

Instructions:

Place the chicken in a zip-top bag and seal it. Whisk together the other ingredients in a small dish and pour over the chicken. Close the bag firmly and gently shake it to thoroughly coat the chicken. Allow chicken to marinate for 25 minutes in the refrigerator, shaking bag lightly twice during this time to recoat chicken. Remove the chicken from the marinade and discard the leftover marinade. Preheat the grill or the oven broiler to medium-high heat. 8–10 minutes each side on the grill or under the broiler, or until the chicken is no more pinkish and the juices are opaque.

Nutritional Values: Calories: 144 kcal /Carbohydrates: 1 g /Protein: 26 g /Fat: 4 g/Sodium: 188 mg

Sun-Dried Tomato Salmon

Total Time: 50 mins / **Prep. Time:** 30 mins /**Cooking Time:** 20 mins /**Difficulty:** Easy /**Serving Size:** 2 servings

Ingredients:

- 2 salmon fillets
- Cooking spray
- ¼ cup sun-dried tomato vinaigrette

Instructions:

Put salmon fillets in a bag and drizzle with vinaigrette. To coat, seal the bag and gently shake it. Refrigerate for 30 minutes after marinating. Preheat the oven to 450°F. Using cooking spray, coat a baking dish. Place the salmon skin side down in the baking dish. Over the fish, pour the marinade. Bake uncovered for 20 minutes or until fish flakes. Remove the skin from each fillet and cut it in half.

Nutritional Values: Calories: 150 kcal /Carbohydrates: 1 g /Protein: 23 g /Fat: 6 g/Sodium: 220 mg

Simple Beef Stir-Fry

Total Time: 20 mins / **Prep. Time:** 5 mins /**Cooking Time:** 15 mins /**Difficulty:** Easy /**Serving Size:** 4 servings

Ingredients:

- Cooking spray
- 16 oz. frozen, mixed vegetables, thawed
- 12 oz. beef tenderloin, cubes
- 3 tbsp. lite teriyaki sauce

Instructions:

Warm a large nonstick skillet over medium heat with cooking spray. Cook the meat tossing often, until the meat is browned (approximately 4–5 minutes). Turn up the heat to high. Combine the veggies and teriyaki sauce in the skillet. Cook, stirring regularly, until the beef is cooked through, and the veggies are crisp-tender (about 4–6 minutes).

Nutritional Values: Calories: 123 kcal /Carbohydrates: 6 g /Protein: 18 g /Fat: 3 g/Sodium: 223 mg

Smoked Tuna Melts

Total Time: 14 mins / **Prep. Time:** 10 mins /**Cooking Time:** 4 mins /**Difficulty:** Easy /**Serving Size:** 4 servings

Ingredients:

- 5 oz. smoked chunk light tuna
- 2 tbsp. reduced-fat mayonnaise
- 1 green onion, finely chopped
- 4 large tomato slices
- 2 whole wheat English muffins, toasted
- 4 slices part-skim mozzarella cheese
- Coarse-ground black pepper

Instructions:

Preheat the oven to 375°F. In a bowl, flake the tuna using a fork. Stir in the mayonnaise and green onion until thoroughly combined. Place a piece of tomato and 1/4 of the tuna mixture on each English muffin half. Season the muffin with salt and pepper, then top with a piece of cheese. Warm it in the oven for 3–4 minutes, or until the cheese melts. Make the tuna combination ahead of time and keep it refrigerated until ready to use.

Nutritional Values: Calories: 164 kcal /Carbohydrates: 16 g /Protein: 16 g /Fat: 4

g/Sodium: 280 mg

Simple Grilled Salmon

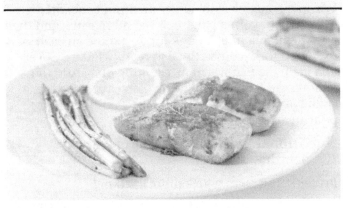

Total Time: 14 mins / **Prep. Time:** 2 mins /**Cooking Time:** 12 mins /**Difficulty:** Easy /**Serving Size:** 1 serving

Ingredients:

- ¼ tsp. olive oil
- Pinch of salt
- Wedge of lemon
- 1 salmon fillet
- Pinch of lemon pepper

Instructions:

Preheat the grill to medium. Rub olive oil all over the salmon, making sure it's uniformly coated. Season the salmon with lemon pepper and salt to taste. Grill the salmon for 6 minutes on each side over medium heat, or until it flakes gently when pricked with a fork. Remove any excess skin. Serve with a squeeze of fresh lemon juice on top.

Nutritional Values: Calories: 141 kcal /Carbohydrates: 1 g /

Protein: 23 g /Fat: 5 g/Sodium: 240 mg

Lemon-Basil Grilled Halibut

Total Time: 15 mins / **Prep. Time:** 5 mins /**Cooking Time:** 10 mins /**Difficulty:** Easy /**Serving Size:** 2 servings

Ingredients:

- 2 halibut fillets
- 1 tbsp. olive oil
- 1 clove minced garlic
- 2 tbsp. fresh lemon juice

- 1/8 tsp. salt
- ½ tsp. dried basil
- 1 tsp. dried parsley
- ¼ tsp. black pepper
- 1/8 tsp. red pepper flakes

Instructions:

Combine olive oil, garlic, lemon juice, salt, basil, parsley, pepper, and red pepper flakes in a mixing bowl. Drizzle the marinade evenly over the halibut in a zip-top plastic bag. Seal the bag and gently shake it to coat the fish. Preheat the grill to medium-high heat. Place the fish on the grill, drizzle with any leftover marinade, and cook for 4–6 minutes per side, or until the fish flakes readily when pierced with a fork.

Nutritional Values: Calories: 161 kcal /Carbohydrates: 2 g /

Protein: 10 g /Fat: 9 g/Sodium: 199 mg

Herb-Grilled Bass

Total Time: 30 mins / **Prep. Time:** 10 mins /**Cooking Time:** 20 mins /**Difficulty:** Easy

Serving Size: 0 servings

Ingredients:

- 2 bass fillets
- ½ tsp. onion powder
- ½ tsp. garlic salt
- ¼ tsp. lemon pepper
- ½ tsp. paprika
- ½ clove minced garlic
- 1 tbsp. reduced-calorie margarine
- ¼ tsp. dried parsley
- Cooking spray

Instructions:

Preheat the grill to medium. Using olive oil cooking spray, lightly coat both sides of the fish fillets. In a small bowl, combine the onion powder, garlic salt, lemon pepper and paprika and whisk well to combine. Season both sides of the fish fillets with the seasoning mixture. Heat the margarine, garlic, with parsley in a skillet over medium heat just before grilling. When the margarine has melted, remove from the heat and cover to keep warm. Cooking spray the grill rack or grill basket. 4–6 minutes per side on the grill, or until salmon flakes easily with a fork.

Drizzle the margarine mixture over the fish.

Nutritional Values: Calories: 133 kcal /Carbohydrates: 1 g /Protein: 21 g /Fat: 5 g/Sodium: 266 mg

Lime Grilled Chicken

Total Time: 20 mins / **Prep. Time:** 5 mins /**Cooking Time:** 15 mins /**Difficulty:** Easy /**Serving Size:** 2 servings

Ingredients:

- 2 skinless chicken breast cutlets
- ¼ cup fresh-squeezed lime juice
- 2 tbsp. chopped, fresh cilantro leaves
- 2 tsp. corn oil
- ½ tsp. chili powder
- 1 tsp. minced garlic
- 2 tsp. grated lime peel

Instructions:

Lime juice, cilantro, oil, garlic, and chili powder should all whisk together in a small bowl. Fill a big zip-top bag halfway with the mixture. Shake well to coat the chicken cutlets. Heat the grill to medium-high. Place the chicken on the grill rack and cook for 15 minutes, or until the juices flow clear when probed with a fork. Remove and discard any leftover marinade. Lime peel should be sprinkled over cooked chicken.

Nutritional Values: Calories: 155 kcal /Carbohydrates: 5 g /Protein: 27 g /Fat: 3 g/Sodium: 77 mg

Apricot Glazed Chicken

Total Time: 30 mins / **Prep. Time:** 5 mins /**Cooking Time:** 25 mins /**Difficulty:** Easy /**Serving Size:** 2 servings

Ingredients:

- Nonstick cooking spray
- ½ tsp. grated fresh ginger
- 2 skinless chicken breasts
- 1 tbsp. rice wine vinegar
- 2 tbsp. Apricot Spread
- 1 tsp. olive oil
- Black pepper, to taste
- ½ tsp. crushed red pepper flakes

Instructions:

Preheat the oven to 375°F. Using nonstick cooking spray, coat a small baking sheet. On the baking sheet, arrange the chicken breasts. With a fork or a tiny whisk, combine the apricot spread, ginger, pepper flakes, vinegar, and olive oil in a small bowl. Spread the mixture equally on the surface of the chicken breasts with a pastry brush or a small spoon. Place in the oven for about 25 minutes, or until the chicken is cooked through. Before serving, season with black pepper.

Nutritional Values: Calories: 215 kcal /Carbohydrates: 19 g /Protein: 19 g /Fat: 7 g/Sodium: 493 mg

Salmon Patties

Total Time: 17 mins / **Prep. Time:** 10 mins /**Cooking Time:** 8 mins /**Difficulty:** Easy /**Serving Size:** 7 servings

Ingredients:

- 12 oz. pink salmon
- ¼ tsp. onion powder
- ¼ cup fine, dry breadcrumbs
- 2 dashes black pepper
- ¼ tsp. garlic powder
- 1 tbsp. skim milk
- 1 egg
- Cooking spray

Instructions:

In a large mixing bowl, place the drained salmon and flake it with a fork. Stir together the onion powder, breadcrumbs, black pepper, garlic powder, egg and milk. Coat a large nonstick pan liberally with cooking spray and heat over medium heat. Shape the salmon mixture into 7 patties, each about 3 inches broad and 1/2 inch thick, using a generous 1/4 cup salmon mixture per patty. Cook salmon for 3–4 minutes, or until the bottom is golden brown. As required, recoat the skillet with cooking spray. Turn patties over carefully with a big spatula and cook for another 3–4 minutes or until light brown and cooked thoroughly.

Nutritional Values: Calories: 96 kcal /Carbohydrates: 3 g /Protein: 12 g /Fat: 4 g/Sodium: 97 mg

Sesame-Ginger Salmon

Total Time: 42 mins / **Prep. Time:** 30 mins /**Cooking Time:** 12 mins /**Difficulty:** Medium/**Serving Size:** 4 servings

Ingredients:

- 1 tbsp. reduced-sodium soy sauce

- 1 tbsp. horseradish mustard
- ¼ cup orange juice
- ½ tsp. ground ginger
- 2 dashes cayenne pepper
- 1 tbsp. honey
- 4 boneless salmon fillets
- 1 tsp. minced garlic
- 1 tsp. toasted sesame seeds

Instructions:

Whisk together the orange juice, soy sauce, mustard, ginger, cayenne pepper, garlic, and honey in a small bowl. Drizzle the marinade evenly over the salmon fillets in a large zip-lock bag. Seal the bag and gently shake it to coat the fish. Marinate for 30 minutes in the refrigerator, rotating once or twice. Preheat the grill to medium high heat. Place the salmon on the grill, keeping the marinade aside. Grill the fish for 6 minutes on each side, or until it flakes readily when pierced with a fork, basting it with the marinade. Bring the rest of the marinade to a boil and cook for 2–3 minutes. Drizzle warm marinade over cooked fish and sprinkle with toasted sesame seeds.

Nutritional Values: Calories: 123 kcal /Carbohydrates: 7 g /Protein: 17 g /Fat: 3 g/Sodium: 324 mg

Steak and Portobello Sandwich

Total Time: 20 mins / **Prep. Time:** 5 mins /**Cooking Time:** 15 mins /**Difficulty:** Medium/**Serving Size:** 4 servings

Ingredients:

- 6 cloves garlic, crushed
- 1½ lb. strip, flank, or skirt steak
- 1 cup balsamic vinegar
- ½ lb. Portobello mushrooms
- olive oil spray
- ½ tsp. salt
- 4 whole-wheat hoagie rolls
- ¼ tsp. freshly ground black pepper

Instructions:

In a small bowl, combine the garlic and balsamic vinegar. Preheat a skillet over high heat. Sear the steak for 2 minutes on a hot skillet. Turn the steaks over and cook for another 2 minutes, or until done to your liking. Remove the pan from the heat and set it aside. Using the olive oil spray, coat the skillet. Cook the mushrooms rotating once, for 5 minutes. Place the mushrooms on a chopping board to cool. Boil the prepared garlic-vinegar mixture for 3 to 4 minutes, until the garlic-vinegar mixture has reduced by half in the pan. Divide the mixture among 4 small dishes and put aside. After slicing the rolls open, spray each side with olive oil spray. In a toaster oven, toast the buns for 1 minute. Thinly slice the meat and the mushrooms. On the bottom half of each bun, place roughly 5 ounces of steak and 3/4 cup of mushrooms. Season the sandwich to taste with salt and pepper. Serve each sandwich with the dipping sauce and the top half of the bun, split in half.

Nutritional Values: Calories: 490 kcal /Carbohydrates: 43 g /Protein: 46 g /Fat: 14 g/Sodium: 690 mg

Coconut Shrimp

Total Time: 20 mins / **Prep. Time:** 8 mins /**Cooking Time:** 12 mins /**Difficulty:** Medium7**Serving Size:** 4 servings

Ingredients:

- 1 lb. large raw shrimp
- 1 tbsp. water
- 2 egg whites, beaten
- ¼ cup unsweetened coconut flakes
- ½ cup whole-wheat breadcrumbs
- ½ tsp. turmeric
- ½ tsp. ground cumin
- 1/8 tsp. salt
- ½ tsp. ground coriander
- nonstick cooking spray

Instructions:

Using paper towels, pat the shrimp dry. In a small dish, mix together the egg whites and the water. In a shallow bowl, combine the coconut, breadcrumbs, cumin, coriander, turmeric, and salt. Dip the shrimp in the egg mixture and then in the panko mixture, allowing the excess to drop back into the bowl. Place the shrimp on a wire rack to cool. Rep the process with the remaining shrimp. In the air fryer basket, arrange the shrimp in a single layer. For 2 seconds, coat the shrimp with nonstick frying spray. Preheat the oven to 400°F and air fry for four minutes. Toss the shrimp around. Air fried the shrimp for 2 to 4 minutes, or till golden brown.

Nutritional Values: Calories: 180 kcal /Carbohydrates: 9 g /Protein: 28 g /Fat: 4 g/Sodium: 230 mg

Teriyaki Chicken

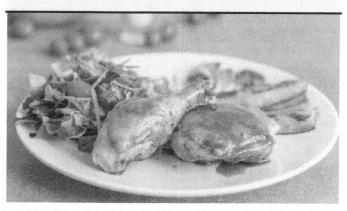

Total Time: 40 mins / **Prep. Time:** 15 mins /**Cooking Time:** 25 mins /**Difficulty:** Medium /**Serving Size:** 4 servings

Ingredients:

- 1 tbsp. corn starch
- ½ cup Splenda granulated sweetener
- 1 tbsp. cold water
- ¼ cup apple cider vinegar
- ½ cup lower sodium soy sauce
- ½ tsp. ground ginger
- 1 clove garlic, minced
- 3 lb. skinless chicken breasts
- ¼ tsp. black pepper

Instructions:

Preheat the oven to 425°F. Using cooking spray, coat a 13" x 9" baking dish. Combine cold water and cornstarch in a saucepan and stir until smooth. Splenda Sweetener, vinegar, soy sauce, ginger, garlic, and pepper are all whisked together in the saucepan. Bring to a low simmer and cook, stirring occasionally, until the sauce thickens and bubbles. Brush teriyaki sauce over the chicken in the prepared baking dish. Brush the chicken again after turning it over. Bake the chicken for 15 minutes in the oven Turn the chicken and bake until the juices flow clear when poked with the tip of a sharp knife. During baking, brush with sauce every 10 minutes.

Nutritional Values: Calories: 170 kcal /Carbohydrates: 3 g /Protein: 30 g /Fat: 3 g/Sodium: 440 mg

Rosemary Chicken

Total Time: 40 mins / **Prep. Time:** 10 mins /**Cooking Time:** 30 mins /**Difficulty:** Medium/**Serving Size:** 2 servings

Ingredients:

- 2 tsp. olive oil
- 1 tbsp. fresh lemon juice
- 1 clove garlic, minced
- 1 tsp. lemon zest
- 1/8 tsp. salt
- 1 tbsp. fresh rosemary, chopped
- 2 chicken breast halves, skinless
- 1/8 tsp. pepper
- nonstick cooking spray
- 1 tbsp. balsamic vinegar
- 3 tbsp. low-sodium barbeque sauce
- 1 tsp. honey

Instructions:

Combine the oil, lemon juice, lemon zest, garlic, salt, rosemary, and pepper in a nonmetallic bowl. Toss in the chicken and flip to coat. Refrigerate for 30 minutes, covered. Using cooking spray, lightly coat the grill rack. Preheat the grill to medium-high temperature. Grill the marinated chicken for 4 to 5 minutes per side, or until the middle is no longer pink. Meanwhile, combine the vinegar, barbecue sauce, and honey in a small pot. Cook the sauce stirring periodically, for 3 to 4 minutes over medium-low heat, or until well cooked. Pour the sauce over the chicken that has been cooked.

Nutritional Values: Calories: 235 kcal /Carbohydrates: 17 g /Protein: 24 g /Fat: 7 g/Sodium: 390 mg

Bourbon's Filet Mignon

Total Time: 15 mins / **Prep. Time:** 5 mins /**Cooking Time:** 10 mins /**Difficulty:** Easy /**Serving Size:** 4 servings

Ingredients:

- ½ tsp. salt
- 4 filet mignon steaks
- ¼ tsp. black pepper
- 2 tbsp. bourbon
- 1/2 cup water with 1 tsp. instant coffee granules
- 2 tsp. Worcestershire sauce

Instructions:

Season both sides of the steak with 1/4 tsp. salt and black pepper and set aside for 15 minutes. In a small bowl, combine the bourbon, coffee mixture, Worcestershire sauce, and 1/4 tsp salt. Heat a big nonstick skillet on high until it is very hot. Cook the steaks for 3 minutes on each side after spraying the skillet with nonstick cooking spray. Reduce the heat to low and cook the steaks for another 2-6 minutes, or until done to your liking. Put them in the oven on separate dinner plates. Bring the coffee mixture to a boil in the skillet over high heat for 2 minutes, or until the sauce is reduced to 2 tablespoons. Distribute the sauce evenly over the steak and serve right away.

Nutritional Values: Calories: 195 kcal /Carbohydrates: 1 g /Protein: 26 g /Fat: 7 g/Sodium: 380 mg

Braised Herbed Chicken

Total Time: 1 hour / **Prep. Time:** 15 mins /**Cooking Time:** 45 mins /**Difficulty:** Medium/**Serving Size:** 4 servings

Ingredients:

- 1 tsp. dried rosemary
- 1 tsp. dried oregano
- 2 cup low sodium chicken broth
- 3 large carrots
- ½ tsp. garlic powder
- 1 tsp. dried thyme
- 1 tbsp. olive oil
- ¼ tsp. black pepper
- 2 cloves garlic
- 1 lb. chicken thighs, skinless
- 12 oz. fingerling potatoes

Instructions:

Combine the thyme, rosemary, garlic powder, oregano, and black pepper in a small bowl. In a Dutch oven, heat the oil over medium-high heat. Sautee the chicken for 3 minutes on each side. Sautee it for 30 seconds more after adding the garlic. In the pan, arrange the carrots and potatoes around the chicken. Over the chicken and potatoes, pour the herb mixture. Bring the chicken broth to a boil in the same pan. Reduce to a low heat, cover, and cook for 30 to 35 minutes.

Nutritional Values: Calories: 260 kcal /Carbohydrates: 23 g /Protein: 21 g /Fat: 9 g/Sodium: 270 mg

Chapter 9: Main Recipes

In a meal with many courses, the prominent or primary dish is called a main course. On most menus, the main dish is the heartiest, heaviest, and most complicated or substantive item. Meat or fish is normally the major element; in vegetarian dinners, the main dish may attempt to imitate a meat course. It's usually followed by a dessert and preceded by a soup, an appetizer, and/or salad.

In this chapter, you'll find several delicious and healthy main recipes for diabetics.

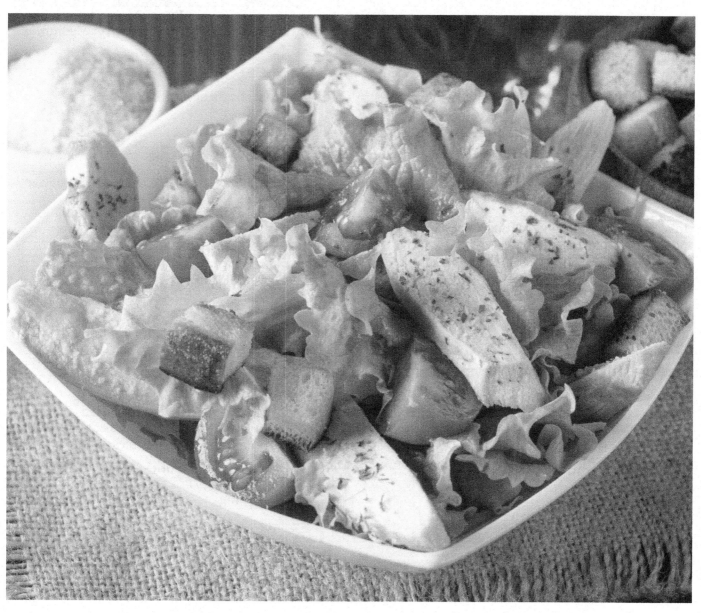

Chicken And Apricot Tagine

Total Time: 40 mins / **Prep. Time:** 5 mins /**Cooking Time:** 35 mins /**Difficulty:** Medium /**Serving Size:** 4 servings

Ingredients:

- 675g boneless chicken chunks
- 1 medium onion, finely chopped
- 1 tsp. ground ginger
- 1 tbsp. olive oil
- 1 tsp. ground coriander
- 1 tsp. cinnamon
- 1 tsp. ground cumin
- 1 tsp. turmeric
- 1 tbsp. tomato puree
- pinch of chilli powder
- 150g dried apricots
- 1 small orange, zested and juiced
- 2 cups chicken stock
- 2 tbsp. fresh coriander, chopped

Instructions:

In a large casserole pot, heat the oil over low heat. Add onions and cook until the onion is tender, then add the ground spices. Stir in the chicken and tomato puree to cover all of the pieces with the spice mixture. After that, add orange juice and zest, chicken stock and dried apricots. Bring to a boil, then lower to a low heat and cover the pan, letting it to gently simmer for 30 minutes, or until the chicken is cooked and the fluids run clear, the sauce has slightly reduced, and the fruits are soft and plump. Season the Tangine to taste with salt and pepper. Before serving, stir in the chopped coriander.

Nutritional Values: Calories: 343 kcal /Carbohydrates: 31 g /Protein: 39 g /Fat: 12 g/Sodium: 444 mg

Chicken Curry

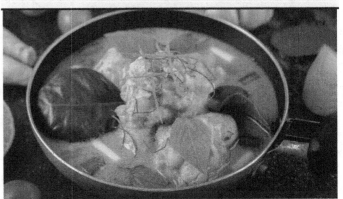

Total Time: 20 mins / **Prep. Time:** 5 mins /**Cooking Time:** 15 mins /**Difficulty:** Medium /**Serving Size:** 4 servings

Ingredients:

- 350g cooked chicken
- 1 pepper
- 5 button mushrooms
- 100g peas, defrosted
- 1 onion
- 1 clove of garlic
- 1 carrot
- 1 tsp. vegetable oil
- 1 cup hot water
- 2 tsp. curry powder
- 1 chicken stock cube
- 1 tbsp. plain flour

Instructions:

Garlic and vegetables should be sliced. In a frying pan, heat the oil and lightly cook the carrot, onions, and garlic. Cook for 2 to 3 minutes with the mushrooms and pepper in the frying pan. Cook for 1 minute, stirring constantly, after adding the flour and curry powder to the pan. Pour the cooked chicken pieces and stock in the pan. Reduce heat to low and simmer for 10 minutes, stirring occasionally.

Nutritional Values: Calories: 244 kcal /Carbohydrates: 12 g /Protein: 27 g /Fat: 8.5 g/Sodium: 400 mg

Garlic And Lime Chicken

Total Time: 4 hours 30 mins / **Prep. Time:** 4 hours /**Cooking Time:** 30 mins /**Difficulty:** Easy /**Serving Size:** 4 servings

Ingredients:

- 4 boneless, chicken breasts

- 1 tbsp. olive oil
- 1 tbsp. fresh lime juice
- salt and black pepper, to taste
- 4 cloves garlic, minced

Instructions:

In a big sealable plastic bag, combine the olive oil, lime juice, and garlic. Toss with a pinch of salt and pepper to taste. Seal the bag after adding the chicken and expelling as much air as possible. Refrigerate the chicken for 4 hours, flipping the bag over once or twice. Preheat oven to 400°F. Remove the chicken from the marinade and discard it. In a roasting tray, arrange the chicken and bake in the oven for 25 to 30 minutes, or until cooked through. Transfer the roasting tray on the grill once the chicken is cooked and grill the chicken for 2 to 3 minutes, or until it begins to crisp up.

Nutritional Values: Calories: 164 kcal /Carbohydrates: 40 g /Protein: 31 g /Fat: 42 g/Sodium: 100 mg

Beef Stew

Total Time: 2 hours mins / **Prep. Time:** 30 mins /**Cooking Time:** 1- 1½ hours /**Difficulty:** Medium/**Serving Size:** 4 servings

Ingredients:

- 1 lb. lean stewing beef, diced
- 2 cups beef stock
- 1 tbsp. vegetable oil
- 5 medium carrots, chopped
- 1½ oz. plain flour
- 1 onion, chopped
- salt and pepper, to taste

Instructions:

In a frying pan, fry the meat on both sides until it is cooked through. After frying the meat remove it from the frying pan and place the meat in a saucepan. Chop the carrots and onions and cook them in a small amount of oil in frying pan. Remove the meat from the frying pan and add it in the saucepan with the meat. Add the flour into the same frying pan and add the stock and seasonings. Give it a good mix. Add this to vegetables and meat and simmer for 1 to 1½ hours, or until the meat is cooked, over a low heat.

Nutritional Values: Calories: 301 kcal /Carbohydrates: 14 g /Protein: 40 g /Fat: 8 g/Sodium: 400 mg

Salmon Fish Cakes

Total Time: 40 mins / **Prep. Time:** 10 mins /**Cooking Time:** 30 mins /**Difficulty:** Easy /**Serving Size:** 4 servings

Ingredients:

- 3 potatoes, diced
- Salt and pepper, to taste
- 1 cup cooked salmon
- 2 tbsp. fresh grated parmesan
- 1tbsp. olive oil
- 1 bunch parsley, chopped
- 4 tbsp. flour
- 1 cup breadcrumbs
- 1 egg, lightly beaten

Instructions:

Peel the potatoes and boil them until they are cooked, then drain and mash. Combine the potatoes, salmon, a pinch of salt and pepper, and half of the parsley in a mixing bowl. Form into round cakes with a mold. Combine the breadcrumbs, parmesan, and the remaining parsley in a mixing bowl. Before rolling the fish cakes in the breadcrumb mixture, coat them in flour and then in beaten egg. In a frying pan, heat the olive oil and gently cook the fish cakes for 4 minutes on each side, or until golden brown. Before serving, remove from the pan and lay on absorbent paper.

Nutritional Values: Calories: 234 kcal /Carbohydrates: 6 g /Protein: 10 g /Fat: 4 g/Sodium: 120 mg

Baked Stuffed Fish

Total Time: 40 mins / **Prep. Time:** 20 mins /**Cooking Time:** 20 mins /**Difficulty:** Medium /**Serving Size:** 4 servings

Ingredients:

- 4 fillets cod
- 1 medium onion, chopped
- ½ cup bread crumbs
- 1 tsp. vegetable oil
- 1 tbsp. fresh parsley, chopped
- ½ tsp. lemon juice
- Salt and pepper, to taste

Instructions:

Preheat oven to 350°F. Prepare the fish by cleaning it. Divide the cod fillets into halves by slicing from in between. In a small bowl, combine breadcrumbs, diced onion, salt, parsley, and pepper. Heat the oil and add it to the crumb mixture. Finally, add some lemon juice. Place 4 fillets, skin side down, on a buttered plate and delicately ladle filling onto each fish. Cover with the remaining four fillets and flatten again. Wrap foil around the dish. Depending on the size and thickness of the fish, bake for 20 minutes. Carefully transfer the fish to a hot serving plate.

Nutritional Values: Calories: 153 kcal /Carbohydrates: 9 g /Protein: 23 g /Fat: 2 g/Sodium: 200 mg

Grilled Cajun Salmon

Total Time: 20 mins / **Prep. Time:** 10 mins /**Cooking Time:** 10 mins /**Difficulty:** Easy /**Serving Size:** 4 servings

Ingredients:

- 4 salmon fillets
- 1 tbsp. Cajun spice mix
- 1 tsp. olive oil

Instructions:

Preheat the grill to medium heat for 10 minutes. Apply a thin layer of olive oil to each salmon fillet. Then add the Cajun seasoning to the fish and marinate for 5 minutes in the fridge. Cook the fish for 8 to 10 minutes over low heat, rotating once or twice. Serve and enjoy.

Nutritional Values: Calories: 186 kcal /Carbohydrates: 0 g /Protein: 20 g /Fat: 12 g/Sodium: 0 mg

Lettuce Wrap Sandwich

Total Time: 10 mins / **Prep. Time:** 10 mins /**Cooking Time:** N/A /**Difficulty:** Easy

Serving Size: 2 servings

Ingredients:

- 8 iceberg lettuce
- 1 tsp. yellow mustard
- 1 tbsp. homemade mayonnaise
- 2 slices ham
- 3 Prosciutto slices
- 5 slices cucumber
- 3 slices chicken breast
- 8 cherry tomatoes, halved
- 1 piece of parchment paper

Instructions:

Place the parchment paper on a cutting board. Lettuce leaves should be placed in the centre of parchment paper, with the sides of the lettuce leaves overlapping and no gap between them. Spread the mustard and mayo first, and then layer the rest of the topping on top. Then add the Prosciutto, ham, cucumber slices, chicken breast, and cherry tomatoes. Using the paper as a basis, roll the lettuce wraps. Make a tight roll with the lettuce wrap. Fold the corners of the wraps towards the centre halfway through folding and keep rolling like a burrito. Roll the remaining paper around the lettuce after it is completely wrapped. Slice the lettuce wrap with a knife and enjoy.

Nutritional Values: Calories: 279 kcal /Carbohydrates: 10 g /Protein: 26 g /Fat: 19 g/Sodium: 1410 mg

Pea Risotto

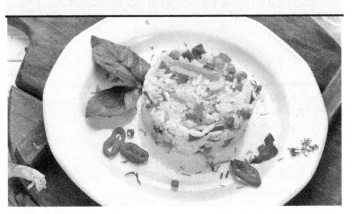

Total Time: 20 mins / **Prep. Time:** 10 mins /**Cooking Time:** 10 mins /**Difficulty:** Medium /**Serving Size:** 4 servings

Ingredients:

- 12½ oz. risotto rice
- 1 clove garlic
- 1 medium onion, chopped
- 1 cup peas, defrosted
- 2 tbsp. olive oil
- 1 vegetable stock cube
- 3 cups boiling water
- 4 oz. cheddar cheese, low-fat

Instructions:

In a medium saucepan, heat the oil and slowly sauté the garlic and onion until tender. Stir in the rice to ensure it absorbs the oil. In a kettle, bring the water to a boil. Gradually pour in some of the water until the rice is covered. Crumble vegetable stock cube in the saucepan. Continue stirring until all of the liquid has been absorbed by the rice. Continue to whisk as you add additional water. Cook until the rice is tender but not mushy, and then add the peas. There should still be some form of sauce on the rice. Cheese should be sprinkled on top and mixed in with the rice.

Nutritional Values: Calories: 167 kcal /Carbohydrates: 14 g /Protein: 10 g /Fat: 8 g/Sodium: 500 mg

Thai Green Chicken Curry

Total Time: 0 mins / **Prep. Time:** 0 mins /**Cooking Time:** 0 mins /**Difficulty:** Easy

Serving Size: 0 servings

Ingredients:

- 1lb. chicken fillets, diced
- 1 medium onion, diced
- 1 tbsp. olive oil
- 1 inch fresh ginger, grated
- 1 garlic clove, chopped finely
- 1 tin coconut milk, low-fat
- 1 tbsp. green curry paste
- 1 lime
- 1 tbsp. tomato puree
- 1 red chilli, diced
- 1 tsp. soy sauce or fish sauce
- 1 cup frozen peas, defrosted

Instructions:

Cook the chicken first. You can either grill the chicken or boil it by adding the chicken breasts in water in a big pan, bringing to a boil, and cooking for 20 to 25 minutes, keeping the chicken plump and juicy. In a wok, heat the oil. Stir in the onion and cook until it is softened. Add the chili, ginger, garlic, and curry paste in the wok. Stir in the coconut milk and tomato puree well. Toss in the peas. Bring to a boil, then reduce to a low heat and continue to cook until the sauce has thickened somewhat. Half the lime, juice and zest one half, and cut the remaining half into wedges. Cook for another ten minutes after adding the prepared chicken, lime juice, and zest.

Nutritional Values: Calories: 244 kcal /Carbohydrates: 12 g /Protein: 27 g /Fat: 8 g/Sodium: 400 mg

Citrus Chicken Skewers

Total Time: 38 mins / **Prep. Time:** 30 mins /**Cooking Time:** 8 mins /**Difficulty:** Medium /**Serving Size:** 6 servings

Ingredients:

- 1/3 cup canola oil
- 1 tsp. grated lemon zest
- ¼ cup orange juice
- 1½ tsp. dried oregano
- 1 tbsp. lemon juice
- 2 cloves garlic, minced
- salt and pepper to taste
- 1 lb. crimini mushrooms
- 4 skinless, chicken breasts, cubes
- 12 cherry tomatoes
- 8 asparagus spears
- 8 grilling skewers

Instructions:

Combine lemon juice, canola oil, orange juice, lemon zest, oregano, salt, pepper, and garlic in a medium mixing bowl. Whisk until all of the ingredients are thoroughly blended. Combine the chicken, asparagus, mushrooms, and tomatoes in a large mixing bowl. Toss until everything is evenly covered. Refrigerate for 20-30 minutes to marinate. On skewers, alternate natively thread chicken and veggies. Remove the marinade and discard it. Meanwhile, preheat the grill to medium. Using tongs, flip skewers once on a lightly greased grill. 5–8 minutes on the grill or until chicken is cooked through.

Nutritional Values: Calories: 240 kcal /Carbohydrates: 7 g /Protein: 20g /Fat: 15 g/Sodium: 100 mg

Walnut-Rosemary Crusted Salmon

Total Time: 20 mins / **Prep. Time:** 10 mins /**Cooking Time:** 10 mins /**Difficulty:** Easy /**Serving Size:** 4 servings

Ingredients:

- 2 tsp. Dijon mustard
- ¼ tsp. lemon zest
- 1 clove garlic, minced
- 1 tsp. chopped fresh rosemary
- 1 tsp. lemon juice
- ½ tsp. kosher salt
- ½ tsp. honey
- 3 tbsp. panko breadcrumbs
- ¼ tsp. crushed red pepper
- 1 tsp. extra-virgin olive oil
- 3 tbsp. finely chopped walnuts
- 1 lb. salmon fillet

- cooking spray

Instructions:

Preheat the oven to 425°F. Using parchment paper, line a large, rimmed baking sheet. In a small bowl, combine mustard, lemon zest, garlic, lemon juice, honey, rosemary, salt, and crushed red pepper. In a separate small bowl, combine the panko, walnuts, and oil. Place the fish on the baking sheet that has been prepared. Apply the mustard mixture to the fish and then top with the panko mixture, pushing it in to adhere. Coat the fish lightly with cooking spray. Bake for 8 to 12 minutes, depending on thickness, until the fish flakes readily with a fork.

Nutritional Values: Calories: 222 kcal /Carbohydrates: 4 g /Protein: 24 g /Fat: 12 g/Sodium: 256 mg

Skillet Lemon Chicken

Total Time: 50 mins / **Prep. Time:** 20 mins /**Cooking Time:** 30 mins /**Difficulty:** Medium/**Serving Size:** 4 servings

Ingredients:

- 3 tbsp. olive oil, divided
- ½ tsp. salt, divided
- 1 lb. boneless, skinless chicken thighs
- 1 lb. baby potatoes, halved lengthwise
- ½ tsp. ground pepper, divided
- 1 large lemon, sliced
- ½ cup low-sodium chicken broth
- 1 tbsp. chopped fresh tarragon
- 4 cloves garlic, minced
- 6 cups baby kale

Instructions:

Preheat the oven to 400°F. In a large cast-iron pan, heat 1 tablespoon oil over medium-high heat. Season the chicken with a quarter teaspoon of salt and pepper. Cook for 5 minutes total, rotating once, until browned on both sides. Place on a platter to cool. In the same pan, add the remaining 2 tbsp. oil, the potatoes, and the remaining 1/4 teaspoon salt and pepper. Cook the potatoes for 3 minutes, cut side down, until golden. Combine the broth, lemon, garlic, and tarragon in a mixing bowl. Toss the chicken back into the pan. Roast the chicken for 15 minutes or until the chicken is cooked properly and the potatoes are soft. Stir in the kale and roast for 3 to 4 minutes, or until it has wilted.

Nutritional Values: Calories: 374 kcal /Carbohydrates: 25 g /Protein: 25 g /Fat: 19 g/Sodium: 377 mg

Chicken Fajitas

Total Time: 40 mins / **Prep. Time:** 20 mins /**Cooking Time:** 20 mins /**Difficulty:** Medium/**Serving Size:** 4 servings

Ingredients:

- 2 tbsp. extra-virgin olive oil
- 1 lb. boneless, skinless chicken breasts
- 2 tsp. ground cumin
- 1 tbsp. chili powder
- ¾ tsp. salt
- 1 tsp. garlic powder
- 1 large yellow bell pepper, sliced
- 1 large red bell pepper, sliced
- 1 tbsp. lime juice
- 1 large onion, sliced

Instructions:

Preheat the oven to 400°F. Using cooking spray, coat a large, rimmed baking sheet. Chicken breasts should be cut in half horizontally, then crosswise into strips. In a large mixing bowl, combine the oil, chili powder, garlic powder, cumin, and salt. Stir in the chicken to coat it in the spice mixture. Stir in the bell peppers and onion until everything is well combined. Spread the chicken and veggies in an equal layer on the prepared baking sheet. Roast for 15 minutes on the center rack. Turn the broiler to high and leave the pan in place. Broil for another 5 minutes or until the chicken is cooked properly and the veggies are browning in places. Remove the dish from the oven. Add the lime juice and mix well.

Nutritional Values: Calories: 357 kcal /Carbohydrates: 32 g /Protein: 30 g /Fat: 12 g/Sodium: 572 mg

Chicken Tenders over Salad

Total Time: 22 mins / **Prep. Time:** 15 mins /**Cooking Time:** 7 mins /**Difficulty:** Easy /**Serving Size:** 4 servings

Ingredients:

- 2 tbsp. all-purpose flour
- ½ cup panko breadcrumbs,
- 1 tbsp. everything bagel seasoning
- 1 large egg
- ¼ cup canola oil
- 1 lb. chicken tenders

- 1 tbsp. white-wine vinegar
- 2 tbsp. olive oil
- 1 tsp. honey
- 1 tsp. Dijon mustard
- 5 oz. mixed baby greens
- 1/8 tsp. ground pepper

Instructions:

In a shallow dish, put the flour, and in another shallow dish, softly whisk the egg. In a third shallow dish, combine breadcrumbs and seasoning. Chicken tenders should be dredged in flour, then egg, and finally breadcrumbs. In a large skillet, heat oil over medium-high heat. Cook it rotating once, until the chicken is golden brown. In a large mixing bowl, combine the vinegar, olive oil, mustard, honey, and pepper. Toss in the greens to coat. Serve the greens with the chicken on top.

Nutritional Values: Calories: 394 kcal /Carbohydrates: 14 g /

Protein: 26 g /Fat: 25 g/Sodium: 337 mg

Chapter 10: Side Recipes

A side dish is any cuisine that is provided as a complement to the main entrée. Aside from this fundamental description, a side dish can take many forms, from basic steamed vegetables to complicated casseroles. Side dishes add variety to a meal's taste profile; and they can also be used to sponge up gravies and sauces.

In this chapter, you'll find several healthy and delicious side dishes recipe for people with type-2 diabetes.

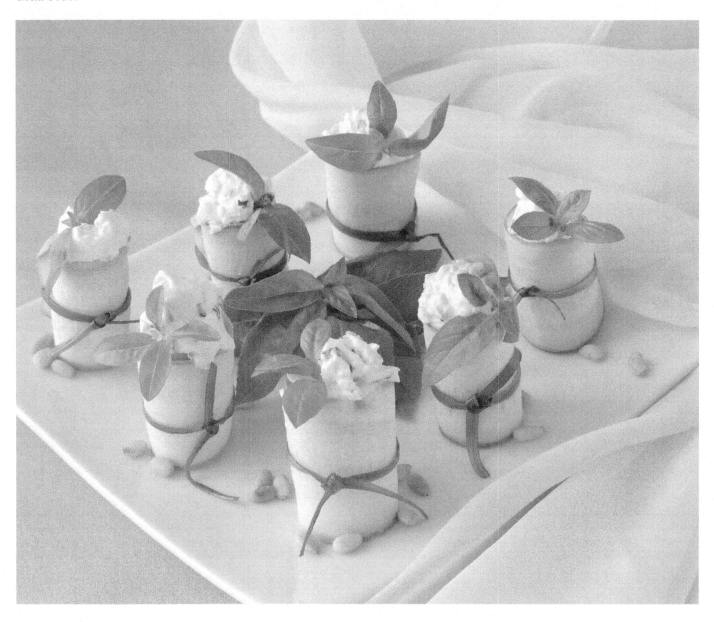

Sautéed Garlic Green Beans

Total Time: 25 mins / **Prep. Time:** 10 mins /**Cooking Time:** 15 mins /**Difficulty:** Easy /**Serving Size:** 6 servings

Ingredients:

- 3-4 cups water
- ½ tsp. salt
- 3-4 chicken broth cubes, low-sodium
- 1 tbsp. olive oil
- 2 lb. fresh green beans
- 2 cloves garlic, minced
- ½ cup red onion, diced
- Salt to taste
- ½ tsp. red pepper flakes
- 2-3 slices fresh lemon
- Pepper to taste
- 2 tsp. lemon zest

Instructions:

Add broth cubes, 1/2 tsp. salt, and green beans to boiling water. Cook the green beans for 7-10 minutes, or until they are barely soft. Pour everything in a bowl and keep aside. Sauté onions in a large pan with 1 tbsp. olive oil until they are transparent. Cook for another 2 minutes after adding the garlic. Mix the green beans with onions, and garlic and season with red pepper flakes, some salt and pepper. Pour green beans into a serving dish and spritz with lemon juice and lemon zest. Serve and enjoy.

Nutritional Values: Calories: 72 kcal /Carbohydrates: 10 g /Protein: 3 g /Fat: 2 g/Sodium: 100 mg

Lemony Steamed Broccoli

Total Time: 21 mins / **Prep. Time:** 15 mins /**Cooking Time:** 6 mins /**Difficulty:** Easy /**Serving Size:** 4 servings

Ingredients:

- 1 lb. broccoli
- 2 tsp. lemon juice
- Salt to taste
- 1 tbsp. butter
- Pinch of black pepper

Instructions:

Broccoli should be divided into florets. Large stems should be discarded. Smaller stems should be trimmed, and stems should be sliced into thin slices. Bring 2 to 3 inches of water and the steamer basket to a boil in a large pot. Cover and add the broccoli and keep it for 6 minutes in the steamer, or until crisp-tender. In a serving bowl, place the broccoli. Toss in the lemon juice and butter to coat gently. Season the broccoli with some pepper and salt to taste.

Nutritional Values: Calories: 59 kcal /Carbohydrates: 6 g /Protein: 3 g /Fat: 3 g/Sodium: 62 mg

Cauliflower Pilaf

Total Time: 20 mins / **Prep. Time:** 10 mins /**Cooking Time:** 10 mins /**Difficulty:** Medium/**Serving Size:** 4 servings

Ingredients:

- 1 large head cauliflower, florets
- 2 tbsp. extra-virgin olive oil
- ¼ cup Italian parsley, chopped
- Sea salt, to taste
- ½ cup golden raisins
- ½ cup vegetable stock
- ½ cup slivered almonds

Instructions:

Process the cauliflower florets in a food processor equipped with a metal blade once they have the texture of rice. Heat the olive oil in a medium pan over medium-high heat and add processed cauliflower in it. Sauté for 2 to 3 minutes, stirring regularly, until the cauliflower softens slightly. Season the cauliflower with salt and pepper after adding the vegetable stock. Reduce to low heat, cover, and simmer for another 5 minutes, or until cauliflower is soft. Remove the pan from the heat and mix in the almonds, raisins, and parsley using a spatula. Serve.

Nutritional Values: Calories: 206 kcal /Carbohydrates: 21 g /Protein: 5 g /Fat: 13 g/Sodium: 237 mg

Herbed Corn On The Cob

Total Time: 10 mins / **Prep. Time:** 5 mins /**Cooking Time:** 5-6 mins /**Difficulty:** Easy /**Serving Size:** 0 servings

Ingredients:

- 1 tbsp. margarine or butter
- 1/8 tsp. salt

- Black pepper to taste
- 1 tsp. mixed dried herbs
- 4 medium ears corn, husks removed

Instructions:

In a small microwave-safe bowl, combine the mixed herbs, butter, salt, and pepper. Microwave for 30 to 45 seconds until butter is melted. Coat the corn with the butter mixture using a pastry brush. Microwave the corn on HIGH for 5 to 6 minutes on a microwavable dish. Serve and enjoy.

Nutritional Values: Calories: 86 kcal /Carbohydrates: 14 g /Protein: 2 g /Fat: 4 g/Sodium: 106 mg

Chutney Glazed Carrots

Total Time: 25 mins / **Prep. Time:** 10 mins /**Cooking Time:** 15 mins /**Difficulty:** Easy /**Serving Size:** 4 servings

Ingredients:

- 2 cups chopped carrots
- 1 tbsp. Dijon mustard
- 3 tbsp. mango or cranberry chutney
- 2 tbsp. chopped pecans, toasted
- 2 tsp. butter

Instructions:

Add carrots with water in a medium saucepan. Over high heat, bring it to a boil. Reduce to medium-low heat and continue to cook for 6 to 8 minutes, or until carrots are soft. Return the carrots to the pot after draining. Cook and stir for 2 minutes over medium heat, or until carrots are coated, adding mustard, chutney, and butter as needed. Just before serving, sprinkle with pecans.

Nutritional Values: Calories: 88 kcal /Carbohydrates: 11 g /Protein: 1 g /Fat: 5 g/Sodium: 151 mg

Carrot Chips

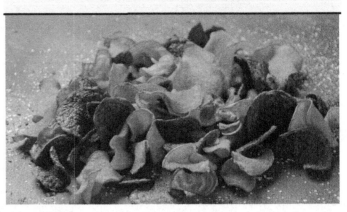

Total Time: 25 mins / **Prep. Time:** 5 mins /**Cooking Time:** 20 mins /**Difficulty:** Easy /**Serving Size:** 2 servings

Ingredients:

- 2 medium carrots, thinly sliced
- 1/3 tsp. salt
- ½ tsp. garlic powder
- 2 tbsp. avocado oil
- ½ tsp. dried parsley

Instructions:

Preheat the oven to 425°F. Set aside a baking sheet lined with foil. Combine the carrot slices with the oil, parsley, garlic powder, and salt in a large mixing bowl until equally covered. Place the carrot slices on the lined baking sheet in a single layer, being careful not to overfill the sheet. Remove from the oven after 20-25 minutes, or until it begins to brown.

Nutritional Values: Calories: 155 kcal /Carbohydrates: 8 g /Protein: 1 g /Fat: 13 g/Sodium: 437 mg

Garlic Bread

Total Time: 28 mins / **Prep. Time:** 10 mins /**Cooking Time:** 18 mins /**Difficulty:** Medium/**Serving Size:** 6 servings

Ingredients:

- 1 cup almond flour
- 2 tbsp. coconut flour
- 1 cup mozzarella cheese, shredded
- 1 large egg
- ½ cup cream cheese
- 1 tsp. garlic powder
- 1 tbsp. butter, melted
- ½ tsp. coarse sea salt
- 1 tsp. dried parsley

- ½ cup fresh grated Parmesan

Instructions:

Set aside a baking sheet lined with parchment paper. Combine the mozzarella cheese, almond flour, and coconut flour in a large mixing dish. Mix the egg and cream cheese into the prepared flour mixture with your fingertips until well incorporated. The dough is going to be quite sticky. Place the dough on a baking sheet lined with parchment paper. Flatten the dough into an 8-inch circle. Pour the melted butter all over the dough and spread it evenly. Parsley, garlic powder, and sea salt should be sprinkled on top of dough. Finish with a sprinkling of Parmesan cheese. Preheat oven to 350°F and bake for 15-18 minutes, or until golden brown. Make 12 strips out of the garlic bread.

Nutritional Values: Calories: 224 kcal /Carbohydrates: 6 g /Protein: 11 g /Fat: 18 g/Sodium: 502 mg

Stuffed Mushrooms

Total Time: 30 mins / **Prep. Time:** 10 mins /**Cooking Time:** 20 mins /**Difficulty:** Medium /**Serving Size:** 6 servings

Ingredients:

- 6 large brown mushrooms
- 2 cloves garlic, minced
- 1 tbsp. olive oil
- 9 oz. cream cheese
- 1 small onion, diced
- 5½ oz. mozzarella, grated
- ½ tsp. pepper
- ½ tsp. salt
- 2 tbsp. fresh chives, chopped

Instructions:

Preheat the oven to 350°F. Trim the thick stems of mushrooms and coarsely chop the stems. In a baking dish, place the mushroom caps. Heat a big frying pan over high heat. Pour in the olive oil. Add the onions after the oil is heated. Once the onions are transparent, add chopped mushroom stems and sauté for another 3 minutes. Now add garlic and cook for 1 minute, or until the garlic is aromatic. Combine the sautéed onions and stems, mozzarella, cream cheese, salt, and pepper in a large mixing dish. Stuff the mixture into the mushroom caps with prepared mixture. Bake the mushrooms for 20 minutes, or until the cheese has melted and turned brown.

Nutritional Values: Calories: 250kcal

/Carbohydrates: 5 g /Protein: 9 g /Fat: 22 g/Sodium: 411 mg

Braised Red Cabbage

Total Time: 2 hours 5 mins / **Prep. Time:** 5 mins /**Cooking Time:** 2 hours /**Difficulty:** Medium/**Serving Size:** 10 servings

Ingredients:

- 15 oz. red cabbage
- 1 cup water
- 1½ cup white vinegar
- 1 tsp. salt
- 1 tbsp. Stevia
- 5 oz. red currant jelly

Instructions:

Cut the cabbage into 1/2 inch strips. Cook the cabbage and Stevia over high heat for 3 minutes. Reduce the heat to low and add water, vinegar, and salt in the cabbage. Allow it to cook for 2 hours, stirring every 30 minutes. Add the jelly after 1 1/2 hours, mix, and continue to cook for another 30 minutes.

Nutritional Values: Calories: 68 kcal /Carbohydrates: 17 g /Protein: 1 g /Fat: 0.1 g/Sodium: 239 mg

Roasted Cauliflower Mash

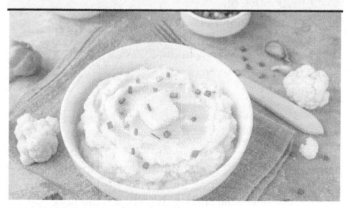

Total Time: 40 mins / **Prep. Time:** 10 mins /**Cooking Time:** 30 mins /**Difficulty:** Medium/**Serving Size:** 4 servings

Ingredients:

- 1 large head cauliflower
- 1 tsp. oregano
- 2 tbsp. olive oil
- 1 tbsp. minced garlic
- 3 tbsp. unsalted butter

- 3 tbsp. sour cream
- Salt and black pepper to taste

Instructions:

Cauliflower should be chopped into florets. Fill a large baking pan halfway with cauliflower florets. Drizzle some olive oil and massage into the cauliflower with your hands. Finally, sprinkle oregano and mix together everything. Preheat oven to 350°F and bake for 25–30 minutes, turning halfway through. When the cauliflower is done, it should be starting to brown. Combine the roasted sour cream, roasted cauliflower, garlic, butter, and salt and pepper to taste in a food processor. Process for 2–4 minutes or until the mixture is smooth and creamy. Stop the processor midway through if required to scrape down the edges. Add extra sour cream if the mixture appears too thick. Place in a serving bowl. Serve with a dollop of butter, chives, and chilli flakes, if preferred.

Nutritional Values: Calories: 188 kcal /Carbohydrates: 13 g /Protein: 5 g /Fat: 14 g/Sodium: 122 mg

Garlic Mushrooms

Total Time: 25 mins / **Prep. Time:** 15 mins /**Cooking Time:** 10 mins /**Difficulty:** Easy /**Serving Size:** 8 servings

Ingredients:

- 1 tbsp. olive oil
- ¼ tsp. black pepper
- 3 cloves garlic, finely chopped
- ½ fresh red chilli, chopped
- 3 tbsp. white wine
- 750g mushrooms, thickly sliced
- 2 tbsp. fresh parsley

Instructions:

In a nonstick frying pan, heat the oil. Fry chilli and garlic in heated oil for 2 minutes. Add mushrooms to the frying pan and cook for 4-5 minutes, or until all liquid has evaporated. Mix the white wine and parsley in the pan and cook for another 2 minutes after seasoning. Serve with your favorite main dish and enjoy.

Nutritional Values: Calories: 35 kcal /Carbohydrates: 0.6 g /Protein: 2.6 g /Fat: 1.6 g/Sodium: 10 mg

Cranberry Sauce

Total Time: 15 mins / **Prep. Time:** 5 mins /**Cooking Time:** 10 mins /**Difficulty:** Easy /**Serving Size:** 8 servings

Ingredients:

- 350g fresh cranberries
- 1 orange juice and grated peel
- sweetener to taste
- 3 tbsp. port

Instructions:

In a pan, combine the port, cranberries, orange peel, and juice. Cover and cook for 8–10 minutes, or until the cranberries are cooked and moist. Add some sweetener according to taste. Cool and refrigerate until you're ready to use it.

Nutritional Values: Calories: 21 kcal /Carbohydrates: 2.5 g /Protein: 0.2 g /Fat: 0 g/Sodium: 0 mg

Savoy Coleslaw

Total Time: 10 mins / **Prep. Time:** 10 mins /**Cooking Time:** N/A /**Difficulty:** Easy

Serving Size: 8 servings

Ingredients:

- 400g cabbage
- 2–3 carrots
- 1 leek
- 1 lemon juice
- 3 tbsp. olive oil
- 1 tsp. grain mustard
- pinch of pepper

Instructions:

Remove any particularly thick stems before slicing the cabbage finely using a mandolin. Grate the carrots and shred the leek finely. Add the vegetables to a mixing bowl. Combine the lemon juice, olive oil, pepper and mustard in a mixing bowl. Mix well and chill for at least one hour before serving.

Nutritional Values: Calories: 68 kcal /Carbohydrates: 4 g /Protein: 1 g /Fat: 4 g/Sodium: 90 mg

Tzatziki

Total Time: 10 mins / **Prep. Time:** 10 mins /**Cooking Time:** N/A /**Difficulty:** Easy

Serving Size: 4 servings

Ingredients:

- ½ cucumber, peeled and grated
- 2 cloves garlic, crushed
- 1 cup Greek yogurt
- 1 tbsp. olive oil
- ¼ tsp. black pepper
- 1 tbsp. fresh mint, chopped

Instructions:

Wrap the cucumber in a clean kitchen towel and squeeze to remove the majority of the liquid. Add it to the mixing bowl after squeezing. Combine the remaining ingredients in mixing bowl and serve.

Nutritional Values: Calories: 69 kcal /Carbohydrates: 3 g /Protein: 7 g /Fat: 3 g/Sodium: 70 mg

Apple and Cranberry Sauce

Total Time: 15 mins / **Prep. Time:** 10 mins /**Cooking Time:** 5 mins /**Difficulty:** Easy /**Serving Size:** 6 servings

Ingredients:

- 2 tbsp. cranberry sauce
- 2 apples
- 1 tbsp. dried cranberries

Instructions:

The apples should be cored and roughly chopped before being added to a pan with a splash of water. Combine the dried cranberries and cranberry sauce in the pan with apples. Heat the sauce gently for 5 minutes, stirring frequently, till the apples have softened.

Nutritional Values: Calories: 41 kcal /Carbohydrates: 9 g /Protein: 0.3 g /Fat: 0.2 g/Sodium: 0 mg

Chapter 11: Salad Recipes

Salad is an essential component of every meal. Healthy salad dishes are an essential part of meals. A diabetic salad is the one that is minimal in carbohydrates and won't induce a blood sugar increase.

A light and refreshing lunch might start with a nice crisp salad. They're simple to prepare at home, and with so many health advantages, eating a serving of leafy greens every day might be one of the most beneficial habits to form. Aside from their inherent crisp texture and pleasant taste, as well as their beautiful smells and colors, eating a substantial quantity of fresh, salad can provide considerable health advantages. It contributes significantly to illness prevention, a healthy weight, and young energy - and who doesn't want a little more of these?

Many of the salads recipes below are also rich in protein, making them hearty enough to serve as a main course. Avocados, almonds, and a low-carb dressing are all good sources of healthy fats in a diabetic salad.

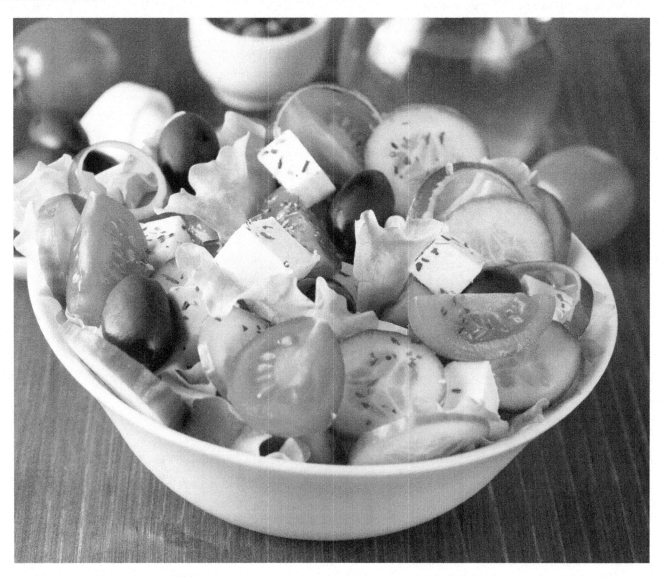

Arugula Artichoke Salad

Total Time: 5 mins / **Prep. Time:** 5 mins /**Cooking Time:** N/A /**Difficulty:** Easy

Serving Size: 1 serving

Ingredients:

- 2 cups arugula
- ½ tsp. Dijon mustard
- 4 pieces artichoke hearts, marinated
- 1 tsp. olive oil
- ½ tsp lemon juice
- 1 tsp. parmesan cheese, grated

Instructions:

Arrange the fresh arugula on a platter. To prepare the dressing, mix together Dijon mustard, olive oil, and lemon juice in a small bowl. Slice artichoke hearts in thin layers on a cutting board. After that, grate the parmesan cheese. Top the salad with sliced artichoke hearts, grated parmesan, and the dressing.

Nutritional Values: Calories: 87 kcal /Carbohydrates: 3 g /Protein: 2 g /Fat: 7 g/Sodium: 254 mg

Chopped Cashew Salad

Total Time: 5 mins / **Prep. Time:** 5 mins /**Cooking Time:** N/A /**Difficulty:** Easy

Serving Size: 1 serving

Ingredients:

- 2 cups salad mix, pre-chopped
- 4 cherry tomatoes
- 20 cashews, non-salted
- Salad dressing of your choice

Instructions:

In a bowl, place the salad mix. Cherry tomatoes and chopped cashews go on top. Toss in your preferred dressing. Serve and enjoy.

Nutritional Values: Calories: 242 kcal /Carbohydrates: 23 g /Protein: 7 g /Fat: 15 g/Sodium: 236 mg

Hemp Hearts Salad

Total Time: 5 mins / **Prep. Time:** 5 mins /**Cooking Time:** N/A /**Difficulty:** Easy

Serving Size: 1 serving

Ingredients:

- 2 cups baby spinach
- ½ cucumber, sliced
- 5 cherry tomatoes, halved
- 3 tbsp. hemp hearts

Instructions:

In a large salad dish, place the spinach. Cucumbers, tomatoes, and hemp hearts go on top. Serve right away.

Nutritional Values: Calories: 225 kcal /Carbohydrates: 9 g /Protein: 12 g /Fat: 15 g/Sodium: 30 mg

Pistachio And Strawberry Spinach Salad

Total Time: 5 mins / **Prep. Time:** 5 mins /**Cooking Time:** N/A /**Difficulty:** Easy

Serving Size: 1 serving

Ingredients:

- 2 cups baby spinach
- 4 strawberries, sliced
- ½ cup shelled pistachios

Instructions:

Toss all of the ingredients together in a bowl and serve right away.

Nutritional Values: Calories: 196 kcal /Carbohydrates: 15 g /Protein: 6 g /Fat: 14 g/Sodium: 65 mg

Heirloom Tomato Salad

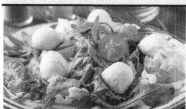

Total Time: 10 mins / **Prep. Time:** 10 mins /**Cooking Time:** N/A /**Difficulty:** Easy

Serving Size: 4 servings

Ingredients:

- 2 large ripe heirloom tomatoes
- 4 leaves of red leaf lettuce
- 1 tbsp. olive oil
- 2 tbsp. pine nuts, toasted
- 1 cup cherry tomatoes
- 1 small clove garlic, mashed
- 1 tbsp. balsamic glaze
- 2 tbsp. basil, thinly sliced
- black pepper, to taste

Instructions:

Arrange four lettuce leaves on four serving dishes. Arrange tomatoes on lettuce in an appealing manner. In a small bowl, whisk together the balsamic glaze, oil, and garlic until incorporated and thick. Drizzle the dressing over the salad. Garnish the salad with pine nuts, basil, and pepper.

Nutritional Values: Calories: 134 kcal /Carbohydrates: 13 g /Protein: 7 g /Fat: 7 g/Sodium: 83 mg

Beet and Blue Salad

Total Time: 10 mins / **Prep. Time:** 10 mins /**Cooking Time:** N/A /**Difficulty:** Easy

Serving Size: 4 servings

Ingredients:

- 6 oz. baby spinach
- ½ cup diced red onions
- 1 cup sliced beets
- ¼ cup balsamic vinegar
- ½ cup carrots, thinly sliced
- 2 tbsp. pure maple syrup
- 2 tbsp. canola oil
- 1/8 tsp. red pepper flakes
- ¼ tsp. salt
- ¼ cup low-fat blue cheese, crumbled

Instructions:

Divide the spinach among four salad dishes evenly. Evenly distribute the onion, beets, and carrots on top. In a small bowl, whisk together the oil, vinegar, salt, maple syrup, and red pepper flakes until smooth and thoroughly combined. Dress the salad with the dressing. Garnish the salad with cheese on top and serve.

Nutritional Values: Calories:234 kcal /Carbohydrates: 6 g /Protein: 12 g /Fat: 7 g/Sodium: 188 mg

Caprese Salad

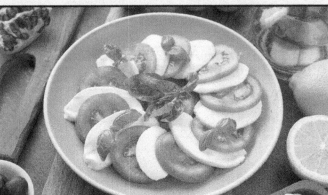

Total Time: 10 mins / **Prep. Time:** 10 mins /**Cooking Time:** N/A /**Difficulty:** Easy

Serving Size: 4 servings

Ingredients:

- 3 medium tomatoes, sliced
- 1/8 tsp. salt
- 2 slices low-fat mozzarella cheese
- 2 tsp. extra-virgin olive oil
- pinch of black pepper
- ¼ cup fresh basil leaves, thinly sliced

Instructions:

Arrange the cheese and tomatoes on the platter, gently overlapping both. Drizzle some oil and season the salad with salt and pepper. Garnish basil on top and enjoy.

Nutritional Values: Calories: 73 kcal /Carbohydrates: 9 g /Protein: 4 g /Fat: 5 g/Sodium: 165 mg

Zucchini Ribbon Salad

Total Time: 15 mins / **Prep. Time:** 15 mins /**Cooking Time:** N/A /**Difficulty:** Easy

Serving Size: 2 servings

Ingredients:

- 2 medium zucchini
- 2 tsp. olive oil
- 2 tbsp. sun-dried tomatoes, chopped
- 1 tsp. white vinegar
- 1 tsp. fresh lemon juice
- 2 tbsp. Parmesan cheese, shredded
- 1/8 tsp. salt
- 1 tbsp. pine nuts, toasted

Instructions:

Use a vegetable peeler and cut zucchini lengthwise into ribbons until seeds are visible. In a medium mixing bowl, combine sun-dried tomatoes and zucchini ribbons. In a small bowl, whisk together the oil, vinegar, lemon juice, and salt until thoroughly combined. Drizzle the dressing over the zucchini and tomatoes and mix lightly to combine. Divide the salad into two serving dishes. Serve with pine nuts and cheese on top. Serve right away.

Nutritional Values: Calories: 133 kcal /Carbohydrates: 9 g /Protein: 5 g /Fat: 10 g/Sodium: 254 mg

Eggplant Caprese Salad

Total Time: 21 mins / **Prep. Time:** 15 mins /**Cooking Time:** 6 mins /**Difficulty:** Easy

Serving Size: 4 servings

Ingredients:

- 2 small eggplants
- ½ tsp. sea salt
- 2 tbsp. olive oil
- 10 oz. mozzarella cheese
- fresh basil leaves, handful
- 2 tsp. sweet balsamic reduction
- 3 ripe tomatoes

Instructions:

Preheat a grill pan to high. While the pan warms up, slice the tomatoes, mozzarella, and eggplants into 1/2-inch-thick rounds. Brush both sides of the eggplant rounds with a thin coat of olive oil, and then season with salt. Arrange the seasoned eggplant rounds in the grill pan that has been preheated. Cook the eggplants for 3 minutes from each side. To make the salad, arrange the mozzarella, eggplant, and tomato slices on a serving plate in an overlapping pattern. Drizzle the balsamic reduction over the top and garnish with chopped fresh basil.

Nutritional Values: Calories: 314 kcal /Carbohydrates: 14 g /Protein: 20 g /Fat: 22 g/Sodium: 728 mg

Purple Cabbage Salad

Total Time: 10 mins / **Prep. Time:** 10 mins /**Cooking Time:** N//A /**Difficulty:** Easy

Serving Size: 4 servings

Ingredients:

- ¾ cup mayonnaise
- ½ tsp. salt
- ½ tsp. apple cider vinegar
- 1½ tsp. Dijon mustard
- 1 tsp. garlic powder
- 1 cup cucumbers, thinly sliced
- 4 cups green and purple cabbage, sliced
- ¼ cup cilantro, chopped
- 2 cups greens, arugula or baby spinach
- ¼ cup fresh basil leaves
- 1 tsp. white and black sesame seeds

Instructions:

To start make the salad dressing combine the mustard, mayonnaise, garlic powder, vinegar, and salt in a mixing bowl and whisk until smooth. Combine the cabbage, cucumbers, selected greens, cilantro, and fresh basil leaves in a large salad bowl. Drizzle the prepared mayonnaise dressing over vegetables and mix thoroughly to incorporate. Serve with white and black sesame seeds as a garnish. You may keep the salad in the fridge for a few hours or serve it right away.

Nutritional Values: Calories: 228 kcal /Carbohydrates: 8 g /Protein: 2 g /Fat: 19 g/Sodium: 260 mg

Oriental Asian Cabbage Salad

Total Time: 10 mins / **Prep. Time:** 10 mins /**Cooking Time:** N/A /**Difficulty:** Easy

Serving Size: 4 servings

Ingredients:

- 2 tbsp. olive oil
- 1 tbsp. white wine vinegar
- 3 tbsp. coconut aminos
- ½ tsp. Garlic powder
- 2 tsp. toasted sesame oil
- ½ tsp. Sea salt
- ¼ cup Sunflower seeds, shelled
- 1 medium Bell pepper, diced
- 14 oz. Coleslaw mix
- 2 medium Green onions, sliced

Instructions:

Whisk together olive oil, coconut aminos, sesame oil, white wine vinegar, garlic powder and salt in a small mixing bowl to prepare the salad dressing. Add the remaining salad ingredients with prepared dressing to coat them. Serve right away or chill for several hours to bring out the flavors.

Nutritional Values: Calories: 120 kcal /Carbohydrates: 8 g /Protein: 2 g /Fat: 9 g/Sodium: 112 mg

Mediterranean Chopped Salad

Total Time: 15 mins / **Prep. Time:** 15 mins /**Cooking Time:** N/A /**Difficulty:** Easy

Serving Size: 4 servings

Ingredients:

- 4-6 cups lettuce, chopped
- ½ medium red onions, diced
- 1 cup cherry tomatoes, halved
- 1 cup Kalamata olives
- fresh parsley, chopped
- 1 cup cucumber, chopped
- ¼ cup feta cheese, chopped
- 2 tbsp. extra virgin olive oil
- 1 tbsp. lemon juice
- Salt and black pepper to taste
- 1 clove of garlic, minced

Instructions:

Combine lettuce, cherry tomatoes, olives and red onions in a large salad bowl. Pour the olive oil and lemon juice into a mason jar. Add the salt, pepper, and garlic whisk. Toss the salad in the dressing well. Parsley and Feta cheese are sprinkled on top. Enjoy.

Nutritional Values: Calories: 93 kcal /Carbohydrates: 8 g /Protein: 3 g /Fat: 6 g/Sodium: 328 mg

Kale Salad

Total Time: 15 mins / **Prep. Time:** 15 mins /**Cooking Time:** N/A /**Difficulty:** Easy

Serving Size: 6 servings

Ingredients:

- ½ cup red bell pepper, chopped
- 3 cups kale, chopped
- ½ cup red onion, chopped
- 3 cups red cabbage, chopped
- 1 cup parsley, chopped
- 1 avocado
- 1 tbsp. lemon juice
- 2/3 cup olive oil
- 2 cloves garlic
- ½ cup water
- ½ cup pine nuts
- Salt and black pepper to taste

Instructions:

Combine red cabbage, kale, bell pepper and red onions in a large salad dish. Pulse chopped avocado, parsley, lemon juice, olive oil, pine nuts, water and garlic in a food processor until smooth. If you want your dressing creamier, use less water. The amount of water you use will determine the consistency you desire. Season the dressing with salt and pepper to taste, and then pour over the salad. Everything should be well combined. Enjoy.

Nutritional Values: Calories: 269 kcal /Carbohydrates: 13 g /Protein: 4 g /Fat: 24 g/Sodium: 44 mg

Avocado Cucumber Tuna Salad

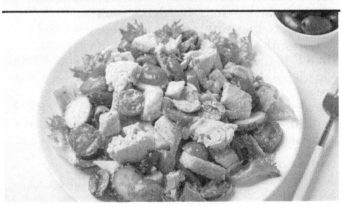

Total Time: 10 mins / **Prep. Time:** 10 mins /**Cooking Time:** N/A /**Difficulty:** Easy

Serving Size: 4 servings

Ingredients:

- 1 ½ cups cucumber, chopped
- 1 cup red bell pepper, chopped
- ½ cup red onions, chopped

- 12 oz. light tuna, drained
- 2 medium avocado, chopped
- 1 tbsp. lemon juice
- 1 tbsp. chives, chopped
- 2 tbsp. olive oil
- Salt and black pepper, to taste

Instructions:

Combine cucumber, bell pepper, red onions, avocado, drained tuna, and chives in a large salad dish. Pour the olive oil, lemon juice, salt, and black pepper into a mason jar. Whisk the dressing and then pour over the salad. Toss to blend salad with dressing and then eat.

Nutritional Values: Calories: 205 kcal /Carbohydrates: 20 g /Protein: 9 g /Fat: 11 g/Sodium: 427 mg

Red Cabbage Kale Salad

Total Time: 10 mins / **Prep. Time:** 10 mins /**Cooking Time:** N/A /**Difficulty:** Easy

Serving Size: 4 servings

Ingredients:

- 3 cups kale, chopped
- 1 tsp Dijon mustard
- 1 small red apple, sliced
- 3 cups red cabbage, chopped
- 3 tbsp. olive oil
- ¼ cup sliced almond
- 1 tbsp. balsamic vinegar
- 1 tbsp. lemon juice
- Salt and pepper, to taste

Instructions:

Combine red cabbage, kale, sliced almond and red apple in a large salad dish. Pour the remaining ingredients into a mason jar. Whisk the dressing and then pour over the salad. Enjoy.

Nutritional Values: Calories: 179 kcal /Carbohydrates: 13 g /Protein: 3 g /Fat: 14 g/Sodium: 92 mg

Chapter 12: Poultry Recipes

Chicken might be a good choice for the ones suffering with type-2 diabetes. Chicken has different type of cuts, all of which are low in fat and high in protein. Chicken may be a great item in your balanced diabetic diet plan if cooked properly. Before cooking the chicken, remove the skin. When feasible, use boneless, skinless chicken breasts. They have less fat than other portions of the chicken.

In this chapter, you'll find several healthy and delicious poultry choices for people with type-2 diabetes.

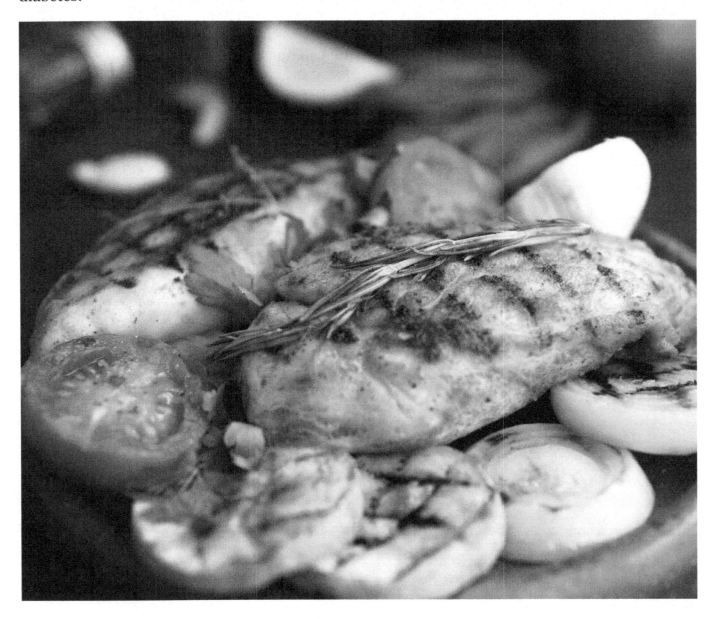

Chipotle Lime Grilled Chicken

Total Time: 1 hour 10 mins / **Prep. Time:** 1 hour /**Cooking Time:** 10 mins /**Difficulty:** Easy /**Serving Size:** 6 servings

Ingredients:

- 6 chicken breasts, boneless
- ¼ cup olive oil, extra virgin
- 1/3 cup lime juice
- 1 tbsp. garlic, minced
- 2 tbsp. cilantro, chopped
- 1 tsp. salt
- 1 tsp. chili powder
- 1 tsp. chipotle pepper powder
- ½ tsp. ground cumin

Instructions:

Combine all ingredients in a gallon Ziploc bag or big covered bowl. Allow to marinate for a minimum of one hour and up to 12 hours. Preheat grill to a medium-high setting. Cook chicken on the grill. Discard any leftover marinade. Cook, flipping periodically, until the chicken is thoroughly cooked through. This should take around 10 minutes, although the duration may vary according to the thickness of the chicken. Serve right away.

Nutritional Values: Calories: 345 kcal /Carbohydrates: 2 g /Protein: 48 g /Fat: 15 g/Sodium: 662 mg

Chili Lime Grilled Chicken

Total Time: 1 hour 15 mins / **Prep. Time:** 1 hour 5 mins /**Cooking Time:** 10 mins /**Difficulty:** Easy /**Serving Size:** 2 servings

Ingredients:

- 2 lb. chicken breasts, trimmed
- ¼ cup lime juice
- ¼ cup olive oil
- 1 tsp. ground coriander
- ½ tsp. onion powder
- ¼ tsp. red pepper flakes
- 1 tbsp. dried basil
- 1 tsp. salt
- ½ tsp. garlic powder
- ¾ tsp. chili powder
- ½ tsp. black pepper

Instructions:

Chicken breasts should be sliced horizontally. This will result in eight thin cutlets that will cook more quickly and evenly. Combine the chicken cutlets and all of the ingredients in a gallon Ziploc bag. Squeeze out any excess air before sealing the bag. Leave one hour for marination. Take each chicken cutlet out of the bag and place on a preheated grill set to medium heat. Grill chicken, rotating periodically, until done. Grilling time is normally between 9 and 10 minutes overall. Serve with side of your choice and enjoy.

Nutritional Values: Calories: 357 kcal /Carbohydrates: 10 g /Protein: 26 g /Fat: 25 g/Sodium: 580 mg

Easy Chicken Curry

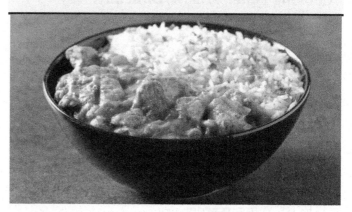

Total Time: 40 mins / **Prep. Time:** 10 mins /**Cooking Time:** 30 mins /**Difficulty:** Medium/**Serving Size:** 4 servings

Ingredients:

- 2 lb. chicken breasts, boneless
- 1 tbsp. curry powder
- 2 tbsp. olive oil, extra virgin
- 1 onion, diced
- 1½ tsp. garlic, minced
- 1 cup coconut milk, unsweetened
- 1 cup chicken stock
- ½ tsp. cayenne pepper
- ¼ tsp. pepper
- 3 tbsp. tomato paste
- ½ tsp. salt
- Green onions, for garnish

Instructions:

In a large pan over medium heat, heat olive oil. To a heated skillet, add chopped onion and minced garlic. Cook until the onion is transparent. Chicken breasts should be cut into tiny, thin strips. In a skillet, add the chicken. Increase the heat to medium high and fry the chicken on both sides. To avoid sticking, stir often. At this time, the chicken does not need to be fully cooked. Once the outside no longer seems raw, you're ready to proceed. Combine the remaining ingredients in the pan. Gently mix. Reduce to a medium-low heat setting. Cover. Cook on low heat for 25-30 minutes. As the sauce simmers, it will thicken. Serve with steamed vegetables, cauliflower rice, or regular rice. Garnish with finely sliced green onion.

Nutritional Values: Calories: 480 kcal /Carbohydrates: 10 g /Protein: 52 g /Fat: 25 g/Sodium: 744 mg

Barbecue Chicken

Total Time: 40 mins / **Prep. Time:** 40 mins /**Cooking Time:** 30 mins /**Difficulty:** Easy

Serving Size: 0 servings

Ingredients:

- 4 chicken breasts
- 1 tbsp. olive oil, extra virgin
- 1/3 cup coconut aminos
- ½ cup ketchup
- 1 tsp. chili powder
- 1 tsp. apple cider vinegar
- 1 tsp. salt
- 1 tsp. ground mustard
- ¼ tsp. onion powder
- ¼ tsp. garlic powder
- ½ tsp. black pepper

Instructions:

Preheat oven to 400°F.In a bowl, add ketchup, apple cider vinegar, coconut aminos, ground mustard, salt, chilli powder, black pepper, onion powder, garlic powder and whisk until completely incorporated. Coat the base of a baking dish with oil. Halve the chicken horizontally to create eight cutlets. In a baking dish, arrange the chicken in a single layer. Spread half of the prepared barbecue sauce on top of the chicken with a spoon, spatula, or brush. Bake the chicken for15 minutes in the oven. Take the chicken out of the oven and turn it over. Spread remaining sauce evenly on top. Continue baking for a further 15 minutes. Serve warm and enjoy.

Nutritional Values: Calories: 349 kcal /Carbohydrates: 13 g /Protein: 49 g /Fat: 10 g/Sodium: 1577 mg

Lemon Herb Roasted Chicken

Total Time: 40 mins / **Prep. Time:** 10 mins /**Cooking Time:** 30 mins /**Difficulty:** Easy /**Serving Size:** 6 servings

Ingredients:

- 10 pieces chicken
- 2 lemons cut into rounds
- 2 tbsp. olive oil, extra virgin
- ¼ cup lemon juice
- ¾ tsp. salt
- 1 tbsp. minced garlic
- 1 tbsp. fresh rosemary, chopped
- ¾ tsp. black pepper
- 1 tbsp. fresh oregano, chopped

Instructions:

Preheat the oven to 450. Spread the chicken evenly on a baking sheet. In a bowl, whisk all marinade ingredients except for the lemon rounds. Stir quickly and pour over the chicken. On the baking sheet, arrange the lemon slices on top of and/or between the chicken pieces. Bake for 30 minutes. Take the oven out of the oven. As you dish the chicken, spoon some of the delicious pan gravy over it and enjoy.

Nutritional Values: Calories: 329 kcal /Carbohydrates: 4 g /Protein: 24 g /Fat: 23 g/Sodium: 380 mg

Italian Shredded Chicken

Total Time: 4 hours 5 mins / **Prep. Time:** 5 mins /**Cooking Time:** 4 hours /**Difficulty:** Easy /**Serving Size:** 6 servings

Ingredients:

- 3 lb. chicken breasts
- ½ cup coconut milk, unsweetened
- 1 cup chicken stock
- 1 tsp. garlic powder
- 12 sun-dried tomato halves, diced
- 1 tsp. dried basil
- 1 tsp. dried oregano
- ¾ tsp. salt
- ½ tsp. onion powder
- 1 tsp. dried parsley
- ½ tsp. crushed red pepper

Instructions:

Chicken breasts should be placed in the bottom of the slow cooker. Add the remaining ingredients on top. Cook on high for 3–4 hours with the lid on. Take out cooked chicken from slow cooker and shred it with a fork. Bring back the shredded chicken to the slow cooker. Stir. Season the shredded chicken with additional salt and pepper to taste. Serve with cauliflower rice, white rice, or vegetables.

Nutritional Values: Calories: 290 kcal /Carbohydrates: 5 g /Protein: 42 g /Fat: 10 g/Sodium: 583 mg

Chipotle Chicken with Green Beans

Total Time: 30 mins / **Prep. Time:** 10 mins /**Cooking Time:** 20 mins /**Difficulty:** Medium7**Serving Size:** 4 servings

Ingredients:

- 2 tbsp. olive oil
- ½ + ¼ tsp. salt
- 1½ lb. chicken breasts, cubed
- ¼ tsp. black pepper
- 4 chipotle peppers
- 12 oz. fresh green beans
- 1 tsp of chipotle sauce
- 1 tsp. garlic, minced
- 3 tbsp. honey
- ½ tsp. chili powder

Instructions:

In a large pan, heat 1 1/2 tbsp. oil to a medium-high heat. When the oil is heated enough, add the chicken pieces. Season the chicken pieces with salt and pepper. Sauté the chicken uncovered, for 3 to 5 minutes, turning periodically. Chicken should be slightly browned. Take the skillet off the heat and set aside. Reduce to a medium heat setting. Green beans and the remaining 1/2 tablespoon oil should be added to the pan. Cover the pan with a lid. Cook it stirring often, for 10-15 minutes. Stir often to prevent the green beans from sticking to the pan. Continue to stir the browned green beans to the surface so that the remaining green beans brown as well. While the green beans are cooking, cut chipotle peppers into smaller pieces. This will allow them to spread them more evenly across the dish after they are placed to the skillet. When the green beans have finished cooking, return the cooked chicken to the skillet along with the chopped chipotle peppers, garlic,

honey, chili powder and salt. Stir. Cook for another 2–3 minutes, or until everything is warmed through and the flavors have melded. Adjust seasoning with additional salt or honey as required. Serve and enjoy.

Nutritional Values: Calories: 342 kcal /Carbohydrates: 22 g /Protein: 38 g /Fat: 12 g/Sodium: 835 mg

Garlic Chicken Cutlets

Total Time: 17 mins / **Prep. Time:** 5 mins /**Cooking Time:** 12 mins /**Difficulty:** Medium /**Serving Size:** 8 servings

Ingredients:

- 2 tbsp. olive oil
- 1½ tsp. salt
- 4 chicken breasts, boneless
- 1 tsp. onion powder
- 1 tsp. garlic powder
- ½ tsp. black pepper
- 1 tsp. dried parsley
- 2 tbsp. garlic, minced
- 1 tbsp. ghee
- 1 cup chicken stock

Instructions:

Chicken breasts should be sliced horizontally. This will result in eight thin cutlets that will cook more quickly and evenly. Combine garlic powder, salt, black pepper and onion powder in a small bowl. Place this seasoning aside. In a large skillet, heat the oil to a medium-high temperature. Once the oil is heated enough, add the cutlets. Season the cutlets' tops with the seasoning mixture. Sauté for approximately 3 minutes each side, or until each side has a slight browning and the chicken is mostly cooked through. Once browned, remove chicken from pan and set aside. Combine the minced garlic and ghee. Sauté for approximately one minute or until garlic is golden. Reduce to a medium heat setting. Combine parsley and chicken stock in a small bowl. Scrape off any chicken parts adhered to the pan's bottom. Bring back the chicken cutlets to the skillet. Cover and heat for approximately 5 minutes, or until chicken is cooked through.

Nutritional Values: Calories: 192 kcal /Carbohydrates: 2 g /Protein: 25 g /Fat: 9 g/Sodium: 611 mg

Chicken in Mushroom Gravy

Total Time: 25 mins / **Prep. Time:** 5 mins /**Cooking Time:** 20 mins /**Difficulty:** Medium/**Serving Size:** 4 servings

Ingredients:

- 2 tbsp. olive oil
- 8 oz. sliced mushrooms
- 1½ lb. chicken breasts, sliced
- ¾ tsp. black pepper
- 1 tsp. salt
- 2 cups chicken stock
- 1 tbsp. garlic, minced
- 1 tbsp. arrowroot flour
- 1 tbsp. fresh parsley, chopped
- ½ tsp. dried thyme
- 3 tbsp. balsamic vinegar
- ½ tbsp. onion powder
- ½ tsp. dried rosemary
- ¼ tsp. paprika
- 1 tbsp. cold water

Instructions:

In a big skillet over medium-high heat, heat 2 tbsp. of oil. Add mushrooms and chicken after the oil is heated. Season it with sea salt and freshly ground pepper. Sauté for 7 to 10 minutes, turning periodically, or until chicken is browned and mushrooms are soft. Add the garlic and sauté for approximately one minute or until garlic is golden. Reduce to a medium heat setting. Combine the balsamic vinegar, chicken stock, thyme, onion powder, rosemary, and paprika in a medium mixing bowl. Add this sauce in the chicken. Cover and simmer for 4 to 5 minutes, or until gravy is well heated. Add fresh parsley and turn off heat to thicken gravy. Combine arrowroot flour and water in a small container. Shake. Pour the mixture into the gravy and whisk until well combined. You'll see the gravy quickly begins to thicken. Serve with side of your choice and enjoy.

Nutritional Values: Calories: 337 kcal /Carbohydrates: 12 g /Protein: 41 g /Fat: 13 g/Sodium: 958 mg

Marinated Grilled Chicken

Total Time: 1 hour mins / **Prep. Time:** 45 mins /**Cooking Time:** 15 mins /**Difficulty:** Easy /**Serving Size:** 4 servings

Ingredients:

- 4 chicken breasts
- ½ cup Coconut Aminos
- ¼ cup balsamic vinegar
- 1 tbsp. dried parsley
- 1 tbsp. garlic, minced
- 1 tbsp. olive oil
- 1 tsp. salt
- 1 tbsp. dried basil
- 1 tsp. onion powder
- 1 tsp. pepper
- 1 tsp. crushed red pepper flakes
- 1 tsp. chili powder

Instructions:

Combine chicken and all ingredients except olive oil in a gallon Ziploc bag or big covered bowl. Flip the chicken occasionally to ensure that the marinade coats all of the chicken. Allow 30 minutes to marinate. Preheat grill to a moderately high setting. Brush marinated chicken using olive oil. Cook chicken on the grill. Remove any leftover marinade. Grill chicken, rotating periodically, until done. Grilling time is normally approximately ten minutes overall, but will vary according on the thickness of the chicken. Serve right away.

Nutritional Values: Calories: 344 kcal /Carbohydrates: 11 g /Protein: 48 g /Fat: 9 g/Sodium: 1237 mg

General Tso's Chicken

Total Time: 10 mins / **Prep. Time:** 5 mins /**Cooking Time:** 5 mins /**Difficulty:** Medium /**Serving Size:** 2 servings

Ingredients:

- 1 tbsp. hoisin sauce
- 1 tbsp. Thai chili sauce
- 2 tbsp. low-sodium soy sauce
- 1 tsp. light brown sugar
- 1 tbsp. ketchup
- Kosher salt to taste
- 2 boneless chicken breasts, cubes
- 1 tbsp. cornstarch
- ½ tsp. white pepper
- 1 clove garlic, minced
- 1 tbsp. peanut oil
- 1 tbsp. dry sherry
- 4 dried red chiles
- 4 scallions, chopped

Instructions:

Combine hoisin sauce, ketchup, Thai chili sauce, brown sugar and soy-sauce in a small mixing bowl. Set aside after thoroughly mixing. Season the cubed chicken with salt and white pepper in a medium mixing dish. Mix in the cornstarch well, then put aside. Over high heat, heat a wok or a big pan. When the pan is heated, add the peanut oil. Stir in the garlic and red chilies for a few seconds and add the chicken and cook for a few minutes. When the chicken begins to become opaque, add the sherry and continue to simmer for another 2-3 minutes. Heat the mixture to a boil, and then add the prepared sauce. Reduce the heat to medium and continue to cook for another minute or two or until the sauce has thickened and chicken is cooked properly. To serve, remove the pan from the heat, discard the red chilies, and toss in the scallions.

Nutritional Values: Calories: 313 kcal /Carbohydrates: 18 g /Protein: 33 g /Fat: 8 g/Sodium: 990 mg

Buffalo Chicken Burgers

Total Time: 22 mins / **Prep. Time:** 10 mins /**Cooking Time:** 12 mins /**Difficulty:** Easy /**Serving Size:** 4 servings

Ingredients:

- 1 lb. ground chicken
- ½ cup finely chopped celery
- ½ cup shredded carrots
- 1 egg, lightly beaten
- 2 scallions, finely chopped
- ¼ cup crumbled blue cheese
- 2 tbsp. hot sauce
- 4 leaves iceberg lettuce

Instructions:

Combine the ground chicken, celery, shredded carrots, egg, hot sauce, scallions, and blue cheese crumbles in a large mixing bowl. Mix until everything is properly combined. Make four patties out of the mixture. Cook the burgers in a pan, on the grill, or under the broiler until done. Put each burger patty on a lettuce leaf, top with your favourite toppings, then roll up to enjoy as a lettuce wrap.

Nutritional Values: Calories: 220 kcal /Carbohydrates: 5 g /Protein: 25 g /Fat: 11 g/Sodium: 536 mg

Carolina Chicken Wings

Total Time: 1 hour 5 mins / **Prep. Time:** 20 mins /**Cooking Time:** 45 mins /**Difficulty:** Medium /**Serving Size:** 14 servings

Ingredients:

- 3 lb. chicken wings
- ¼ tsp. cayenne pepper
- ½ cup flour
- 2½ tsp. Old Bay seasoning, divided
- ¼ tsp. black pepper
- 2 tbsp. unsalted butter, melted
- ½ tsp. salt
- 1 tbsp. cider vinegar
- 4 tbsp. hot sauce
- 1 tbsp. Worcestershire sauce

Instructions:

Preheat the oven to 425°F. Prepare baking pans by lining them with parchment paper. Combine the cayenne, flour, 1/2 tsp. Old Bay, black pepper, and salt in a gallon-sized plastic bag. Add the wings in batches to the bag and mix until completely covered in flour. Shake off any surplus, and then arrange the wings on the prepared baking pans in a single layer. The wings should not be in contact with each other. Bake the wings in preheated oven for 25 minutes. Bake for another 20 minutes, or until the wings are browned, after turning them with tongs. Combine the hot sauce, melted butter, Worcestershire, cider vinegar, and the remaining 2 tsp. of Old Bay in a small bowl while the wings are baking. Remove the wings from the oven after they've done cooking and coat both sides with the sauce.

Nutritional Values: Calories: 247 kcal /Carbohydrates: 3 g /Protein: 18 g /Fat: 18 g/Sodium: 204 mg

Chicken Meatballs

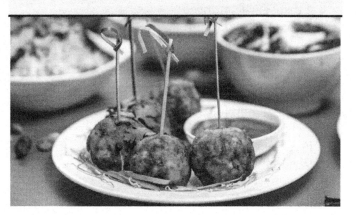

Total Time: 35 mins / **Prep. Time:** 5 mins /**Cooking Time:** 30 mins /**Difficulty:** Easy /**Serving Size:** 4 servings

Ingredients:

- 1½ lb. ground chicken
- ½ tsp. salt
- ½ tsp. garlic powder
- black pepper to taste
- ½ tsp. onion powder
- 1 tsp. Italian season
- 1 tbsp. olive oil
- 1 tsp. flax seed powder
- ¼ cup grated Parmesan
- 1 egg

Instructions:

Preheat the oven to 400°F and line a baking pan with silicone baking sheets or tin foil. Grease the pan and leave it aside. In a large mixing dish, combine all of the ingredients. Combine until all of the ingredients are fully incorporated, then set aside for 5 minutes to cool. Roll the mixture into 12 meatballs and place them on the baking pan when it has rested. Bake the meatballs for 30 minutes, or until slightly browned and cooked through.

Nutritional Values: Calories: 344 kcal /Carbohydrates: 1 g /Protein: 34 g /Fat: 23 g/Sodium: 445 mg

Yogurt Marinated Chicken Breast

Total Time: 50 mins / **Prep. Time:** 10 mins /**Cooking Time:** 40 mins /**Difficulty:** Easy /**Serving Size:** 4 servings

Ingredients:

- 4 skinless chicken breasts
- 2 tbsp. garlic, minced
- 1½ cups Greek yogurt
- 1 tsp. black pepper
- 1 tsp. sea salt
- 1½ tsp. ground cumin
- 1 tsp. paprika
- 1 tbsp. lemon juice
- ½ tsp. chili powder
- Fresh parsley, for garnish
- ½ cup fresh herbs, chopped
- Lemon wedges, for serving

Instructions:

Combine the yogurt, spices, garlic, fresh herbs and lemon juice in a large mixing bowl. Mix thoroughly. Place the chicken breasts in a baking dish that is large enough to hold them tightly. Pour the prepared marinade mixture all over the chicken, making sure it is completely covered on both sides. Grill the chicken for 35–40 minutes over high heat, rotating once, until cooked through. Remove the grilled chicken from the heat and place it on a serving plate. Cover with foil for 10 minutes to allow the meat to rest. Serve with lemon wedges and finely chopped parsley.

Nutritional Values: Calories: 195 kcal /Carbohydrates: 4 g /Protein: 40 g /Fat: 2 g/Sodium: 611 mg

Smoky Whole Chicken

Total Time: 41 mins / **Prep. Time:** 20 mins /**Cooking Time:** 21 mins /**Difficulty:** Medium /**Serving Size:** 6 servings

Ingredients:

- 2 tbsp. extra-virgin olive oil
- 1½ tsp. smoked paprika
- 1 tbsp. kosher salt
- ¼ tsp. cayenne pepper
- 1 tsp. black pepper
- 1 large lemon, halved
- 1 whole chicken
- 1 large onion, wedges
- 6 garlic cloves, crushed
- 2 large carrots, quartered
- 1 cup chicken broth
- 2 celery stalks, quartered

Instructions:

Combine the salt, olive oil, pepper, paprika, and cayenne in a small bowl. Place the chicken on a chopping board and spread the olive oil and spice mixture all over it, including beneath the skin. Fill the cavity with the garlic cloves, lemon halves, and 4 onion wedges. Fill the electric pressure cooker halfway with broth and add the carrots, other 4 onion wedges and celery. On top of the vegetables, place a wire rack or trivet. Place the chicken on the rack, breast-side up. Close and lock the pressure cooker's lid, making that the valve is set to "Sealing." Cook for 21 minutes on high pressure. When the cooking is finished, press Cancel and let the pressure naturally drop for 15 minutes. Turn the valve to "Venting" after 15 minutes to quickly discharge any leftover pressure. Unlock and remove the cover after the pin has dropped. Transfer the chicken to a clean chopping board with care. Remove the skin off the chicken and chop it into desired pieces.

Nutritional Values: Calories: 255 kcal /Carbohydrates: 7 g /Protein: 27 g /Fat: 13 g/Sodium: 578 mg

Chicken Cashew Stir-Fry

Total Time: 30 mins / **Prep. Time:** 15 mins /**Cooking Time:** 15 mins /**Difficulty:** Medium /**Serving Size:** 4 servings

Ingredients:

- 1 lb. chicken breasts, strips
- ½ tsp. red pepper flakes
- 4 tbsp. low-sodium soy sauce, divided
- 2 tbsp. olive oil, divided
- 3 tbsp. raw cashews
- 1½ tbsp. fresh ginger, minced
- 5 garlic cloves, minced
- ½ cup orange juice
- 2 medium carrots, thin strips
- 1 large red bell pepper, strips
- 4 scallions, sliced

Instructions:

Combine 2 tbsp. soy sauce, red pepper flakes and chicken strips in a medium mixing bowl. Toast the cashews in a small dry nonstick pan for 3 to 4 minutes, tossing often, until lightly toasted. Allow to cool after removing from the heat. In a wok, heat 1 tbsp. of olive oil over medium-high heat. Add the ginger and garlic once the pan is heated, and stir-fry for about a minute, or until fragrant. Add marinated chicken to the wok and stir-fry for 3 to 4 minutes, or until the chicken is no longer pink. Set aside the contents of the wok on a plate or in a dish. Toss in the remaining olive oil in the wok. Stir in the carrots and red bell pepper and cook for 3 minutes, or until the vegetables are cooked but still crisp. Cook for another 2 minutes after adding half of the scallions. Return the chicken to the wok. In a small dish, combine the orange juice and the remaining 2 tbsp. of soy sauce, and then pour into the wok. Increase the heat to high and bring the mixture to a boil, stirring frequently. Allow 30 seconds for the contents to boil before removing the wok from the heat. Serve with the cashews and remaining scallions as a garnish.

Nutritional Values: Calories: 304 kcal /Carbohydrates: 16 g /Protein: 30 g /Fat: 13 g/Sodium: 634 mg

Chicken Masala

Total Time: 2 hour 45 mins / **Prep. Time:** 2 hours 5 mins /**Cooking Time:** 40 mins /**Difficulty:** Medium /**Serving Size:** 4 servings

Ingredients:

- 1 cup plain nonfat yogurt
- 2 tbsp. olive oil
- ¼ cup fresh cilantro, chopped
- 1 tsp. Kosher salt
- 1 tbsp. garam masala
- 1½ lb. chicken breasts
- 1 large garlic clove, minced
- 1 small onion, sliced

Instructions:

Combine the cilantro, yogurt, garam masala, olive oil, salt, and garlic in a small bowl. Mix until everything is properly combined. Place the chicken breasts in a gallon bag after dipping them in the yoghurt mixture. Remove as much air trapped before sealing the bag, and then pour the remaining yoghurt mixture over the chicken. Squeeze the contents of the bag to ensure that the yoghurt is evenly distributed over all sides of the chicken. Place the bag in the fridge for at least 2 hours to marinate. Preheat the baking oven to 400°F. On a baking sheet, spread the sliced onion in a thin layer. Carefully remove the marinated chicken from the bag so that the marinade does not spill. Arrange the chicken breasts over the onion slices, spacing them apart so they don't touch. Bake the chicken for about 40 minutes, or until thoroughly cooked through.

Nutritional Values: Calories: 324 kcal /Carbohydrates: 15 g /Protein: 44 g /Fat: 8 g/Sodium: 424 mg

Chicken Scaloppini

Total Time: 30 mins / **Prep. Time:** 15 mins /**Cooking Time:** 15 mins /**Difficulty:** Medium/**Serving Size:** 4 servings

Ingredients:

- 2 chicken breasts
- 4 oz. whole wheat spaghetti
- 2 tbsp. olive oil
- 1/3 cup white wheat
- 2 tbsp. fresh lemon juice
- 3 tbsp. butter
- 2 tsp. capers
- 2 lemon, sliced

- 1 tbsp. fresh parsley, chopped
- pinch of salt

Instructions:

Follow the package directions for cooking the pasta. Slice the chicken breast in half with the knife perpendicular to the cutting board, resulting in extremely thin and broad pieces. Pound each piece of chicken among two wax paper slices until it is 1/4 inches thick. Using flour, coat each piece of chicken. Heat 2 tbsp. butter, 1 tbsp. olive oil, and a pinch of sea salt in a large pan over medium-high heat. When the pan is hot, add the coated chicken and fry it on both sides until thoroughly done. Place the cooked chicken on a platter and set aside to keep warm. In the same skillet, add the remaining tbsp. of butter, olive oil, and salt. Add in the lemon juice and capers and cook for 2 minutes. Divide the chicken, pasta, and sauce between four serving dishes to serve. Serve with lemon slices and parsley as garnish.

Nutritional Values: Calories: 378 kcal /Carbohydrates: 26 g /Protein: 31 g /Fat: 17 g/Sodium: 278 mg

Curried Chicken Skillet

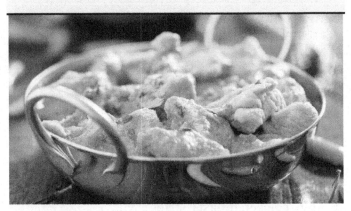

Total Time: 35 mins / **Prep. Time:** 10 mins /**Cooking Time:** 25 mins /**Difficulty:** Medium/**Serving Size:** 4 servings

Ingredients:

- ½ cup +1-1/3 cups low-sodium chicken broth, divided
- 1 tbsp. canola oil
- 2/3 cup quinoa, rinsed
- 1 medium onion, chopped
- 1 medium sweet potato, diced
- 1 cup frozen peas
- 1 celery rib, chopped
- 1 tsp. minced fresh gingerroot
- 2 garlic cloves, minced
- ¼ tsp. salt
- 3 tsp. curry powder
- 2 cups shredded cooked chicken

Instructions:

Bring 1-1/3 cup broth to a boil in a small saucepan. Toss in the quinoa. Reduce heat to low and cook, covered, for 12-15 minutes, or until liquid is absorbed. Cook sweet potato, onion, and celery in a large pan over medium-high heat until potatoes are cooked, about 10-12 minutes. Cook and stir for 2 minutes with peas, garlic, ginger, and spices. Heat through the chicken and add the remaining broth. Add the quinoa and mix well.

Nutritional Values: Calories: 367 kcal /Carbohydrates: 39 g /Protein: 29 g /Fat: 11 g/Sodium: 450 mg

Chapter 13: Seafood Recipes

Seafood can be beneficial to diabetics if consumed in the appropriate quantity and variety, depending on your diabetes type. These can help you regulate your blood sugar, lower your risk of heart disease, and deliver protein. Seafood, fish, and shellfish such as lobsters and crabs may also help in the management of diabetes. Diabetes mellitus nerve involvement can be reduced by eating seafood.

Seafood is an excellent source of proteins, energy, acids, minerals, and vitamins, which will help you stay healthy if you have diabetes.

In this chapter, you'll find several healthy and delicious seafood choices for people with type-2 diabetes.

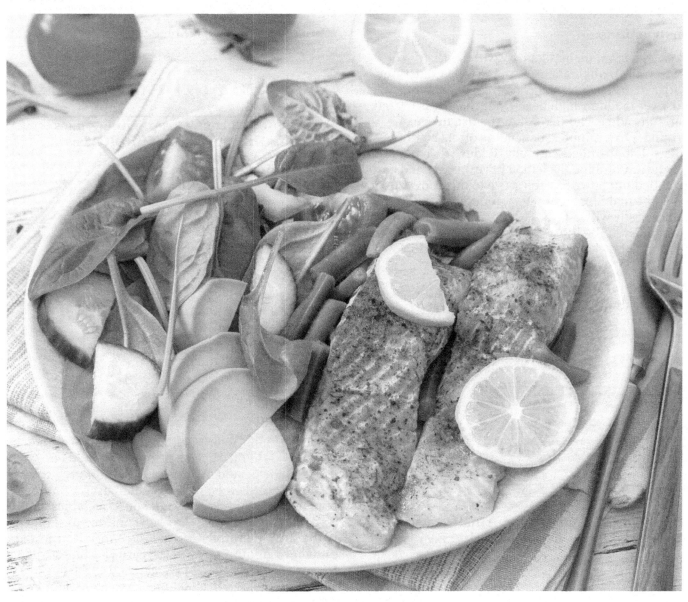

Lemon Butter Mahi Mahi

Total Time: 15 mins / **Prep. Time:** 5 mins
/**Cooking Time:** 10 mins /**Difficulty:** Easy
/**Serving Size:** 4 servings

Ingredients:

- 4 mahi mahi fillets
- ½ tsp. black pepper
- ½ tsp. salt
- ¼ cup vegan butter
- 2 tbsp. olive oil, extra virgin
- 2 tbsp. lemon juice
- 2 tbsp. fresh parsley, finely chopped
- 2 tsp. garlic, minced

Instructions:

Press the mahi mahi fillets dry with paper towels. Season the mahi mahi on both the top and bottom with salt and pepper. In a large skillet heat the oil, over medium-high heat. Once the pan is heated, carefully add each fillet. Allow the fish to cook for around 4 to 5 minutes, depending on size of the fillets. Flip the fillets carefully. Reduce to a medium-low heat. Combine the lemon juice, butter, and garlic in a medium bowl. Stir the sauce to mix. Cover and cook the mahi mahi for 3 to 4 minutes or until it flakes easily with a fork. Turn off the heat and remove the skillet off the heat. Combine the parsley and sauce in a small bowl and ladle the sauce all over the mahi mahi.

Nutritional Values: Calories: 313 kcal /Carbohydrates: 1 g /Protein: 32 g /Fat: 20 g/Sodium: 543 mg

Lemon Butter Shrimp

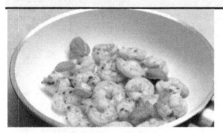

Total Time: 10 mins / **Prep. Time:** 5 mins /**Cooking Time:** 5 mins /**Difficulty:** Easy

Serving Size: 4 servings

Ingredients:

- ¼ cup butter
- ½ tsp. salt

- 1 lb. shrimp
- 2 tbsp. lemon juice
- 2 tsp. parsley, chopped
- ¼ tsp. pepper
- 1 tbsp. garlic

Instructions:

Season the shrimps with salt and freshly ground pepper. On a medium heat, melt butter in a skillet. Add seasoned shrimps to the skillet after the butter has melted. Cook for 3–5 minutes, stirring periodically, or until shrimp is pink. Increase the heat to medium-high. Combine minced garlic and lemon juice in a small bowl. Stir for 1 minute at a low heat. Garnish with parsley and s Serve immediately with zoodles, spaghetti, or roasted vegetables.

Nutritional Values: Calories: 217 kcal /Carbohydrates: 1 g /Protein: 23 g /Fat: 13 g/Sodium: 1172 mg

Garlic Shrimp Stir Fry

Total Time: 20 mins / **Prep. Time:** 5 mins /**Cooking Time:** 15 mins /**Difficulty:** Easy /**Serving Size:** 4 servings

Ingredients:

- 1½ tbsp. olive oil
- 1 bell pepper, thinly sliced
- 12 oz. green beans
- 1/3 cup coconut aminos
- 1 tbsp. garlic, minced
- ¼ + ¼ tsp. salt
- ¼ tsp. black pepper
- 1 tsp. sesame oil
- 1 lb. shrimp, peeled and deveined
- ¼ tsp. ground ginger
- ¼ tsp. garlic powder
- Parsley chopped, for garnish

Instructions:

In a large skillet over medium-high heat, heat the olive oil. Add the sliced bell pepper and green beans to the heated oil. Cook for 5–7 minutes, tossing regularly, until green beans begin to brown but remain crisp. You do not want your vegetables to be soft at this point, since they will continue to simmer in the shrimp broth later. Add the minced garlic and sauté for 1 minute, or until the garlic becomes golden. Season shrimp with pepper, salt, and garlic powder while vegetables are sautéing. Place aside. Combine sesame oil, 1/4 tsp. salt, ground ginger and coconut aminos in a pan along with the vegetables. Stir. Add the shrimp that have been seasoned. Cook, covered, for 3–4 minutes, or until shrimp is pink. Garnish with fresh parsley, chopped and serve.

Nutritional Values: Calories: 229 kcal /Carbohydrates: 13 g /Protein: 25 g /Fat: 8 g/Sodium: 1211 mg

Chipotle Lime Salmon

Total Time: 14 mins / **Prep. Time:** 5 mins /**Cooking Time:** 9 mins /**Difficulty:** Medium /**Serving Size:** 4 servings

Ingredients:

- 4 salmon fillets
- ¾ tsp. chipotle chile pepper
- 1 tbsp. olive oil
- ½ tsp. black pepper
- ½ tsp. salt
- 2 tbsp. lime juice
- ¼ cup butter
- 2 tsp. garlic, minced
- 1 tbsp. fresh parsley, chopped

Instructions:

In a large pan over medium-high heat, heat the olive oil. Use the paper towels to pat the salmon dry. Season the top of the salmon with salt, chipotle chilli pepper and black pepper. Press the spices into the fish gently. When the oil is heated, put the salmon in the skillet skin side up. Sauté for 4–5 minutes or until the portion of the salmon that touches the pan develops a golden brown crust. Flip the salmon carefully so that the skin side is now facing down. In a pan, add lime juice, butter and chopped garlic. Continue sautéing for an additional 3 to 4 minutes or until salmon is opaque. When ready to serve, garnish parsley over the salmon and serve with sides of your choice.

Nutritional Values: Calories: 376 kcal /Carbohydrates: 1 g /Protein: 34 g /Fat: 26 g/Sodium: 382 mg

Greek Shrimp and Broccoli

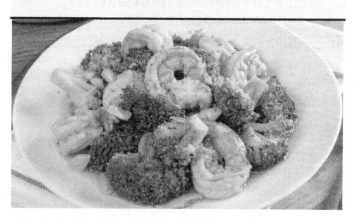

Total Time: 25 mins / **Prep. Time:** 5 mins /**Cooking Time:** 20 mins /**Difficulty:** Easy /**Serving Size:** 4 servings

Ingredients:

- 16 oz. fresh broccoli florets
- ½ + ¼ tsp. salt
- ¼ + ¼ tsp. garlic powder
- 1½ + 1 tbsp. olive oil
- 1 lb. shrimp, peeled and deveined
- ½ tsp. dried oregano
- 1 tbsp. lemon juice
- ¼ tsp. garlic powder
- ½ tsp. dried basil
- ¼ tsp. onion powder

Instructions:

Preheat oven to 425°F. On a baking sheet, spread broccoli florets in a layer. Drizzle 1 1/2 tbsp. olive oil, season with ½ tsp. salt, and sprinkle ¼ tsp. garlic powder all over the broccoli. Roast it for 15 minutes in the oven. Meanwhile, combine shrimp, 1 tbsp. olive oil, oregano, lemon juice, ¼ tsp. garlic powder, basil, onion powder, and ¼ tsp. salt in a mixing bowl. After 15 minutes, take broccoli from oven and place shrimp in a uniform layer on the pan with the vegetables and bake for 5–7 minutes in the oven.

Nutritional Values: Calories: 233 kcal /Carbohydrates: 8 g /Protein: 26 g /Fat: 11 g/Sodium: 355 mg

Seafood Parcels

Total Time: 35 mins / **Prep. Time:** 15 mins /**Cooking Time:** 20 mins /**Difficulty:** Easy /**Serving Size:** 2 servings

Ingredients:

- 160g broccoli florets
- 100g Pollock, cut into 2 chunks
- 100g salmon, cubed
- 50g prawns
- 1 red pepper, cut into strips
- 6 spring onions, sliced
- 10g parsley
- 1 tbsp. lemon juice
- 2 tbsp. water
- black pepper
- Lemon wedges to serve
- 2 tsp. olive oil

Instructions:

Preheat the oven to 400°Fand blanch the broccoli in boiling water for 3–4 minutes before draining. Divide the fish, seafood, and vegetables evenly between two squares of foil. Add the parsley and a generous dash of pepper to taste. Add the olive oil and water after squeezing the lemon over each. To form a parcel, fold the foil into the centre, then place on a baking pan and bake for 15 minutes. Each parcel should be served with a lemon slice.

Nutritional Values: Calories: 257 kcal /Carbohydrates: 8 g /Protein: 27 g /Fat: 12 g/Sodium: 310 mg

Squid and Prawn Skewers

Total Time: 20 mins / **Prep. Time:** 15 mins /**Cooking Time:** 5 mins /**Difficulty:** Easy /**Serving Size:** 10 servings

Ingredients:

- 300g raw squid rings
- 1 clove garlic, crushed
- 165g raw peeled jumbo king prawns
- 1 lemon juice + zest
- 1 small red chilli, finely chopped
- 1 tsp. rapeseed oil

Instructions:

Combine the prawns and squid with the garlic, lemon juice, chilli, and zest, leaving a small amount of the zest for garnish. Allow for a 5-minute marinating time. On each skewer, thread a squid ring, a prawn, then another squid ring. In a large nonstick frying pan, heat the oil and cook the skewers, flipping once, until the prawns are thoroughly cooked.

Nutritional Values: Calories: 42 kcal /Carbohydrates: 0.1 g /Protein: 7 g /Fat: 1 g/Sodium: 170 mg

Salmon On Fennel Ratatouille

Total Time: 25 mins / **Prep. Time:** 10 mins /**Cooking Time:** 15 mins /**Difficulty:** Medium /**Serving Size:** 1 servings

Ingredients:

- 1tsp. olive oil
- 1 yellow pepper, chopped
- 1 small red onion, chopped
- pinch of dried oregano
- 1 clove garlic, crushed
- 2 fresh ripe tomatoes, chopped
- pinch of pepper
- 1 salmon fillet
- ½ head of fennel, thinly sliced
- 2 tbsp. water
- fresh basil leaves, to serve

Instructions:

In a large skillet, heat the oil over medium heat. Stir in the onion for 2–3 minutes, until it softens. Add the chopped yellow pepper and continue to stir for another 3–4 minutes. Add the oregano, garlic, tomatoes, seasoning, and fennel in skillet and stir for another 2 minutes before bringing to a simmer. Put the salmon on top of the prepared ratatouille, cover with a lid or foil, and heat it up. Cook it for 4–5 minutes, or until the fish is fully cooked. Remove the salmon from the pan and add a few chopped fresh basil leaves to the ratatouille before serving.

Nutritional Values: Calories: 421 kcal /Carbohydrates: 20 g /Protein: 29 g /Fat: 22 g/Sodium: 180 mg

Poached Salmon Blinis

Total Time: 25 mins / **Prep. Time:** 15 mins
/**Cooking Time:** 10 mins /**Difficulty:** Medium
/**Serving Size:** 16 servings

Ingredients:

- 2 salmon steaks
- 1 tbsp. low-fat yogurt
- 100g watercress
- 1 pack 16 blinis
- 1 lemon juice and zest
- 1 tbsp. cream cheese, low-fat
- fresh dill, to garnish
- salad leaves, to garnish
- lemon wedges, to garnish

Instructions:

In a small saucepan, place the salmon steaks, cover with boiling water, and cook for 5 minutes, covered. Turn off the heat and let the salmon sit for 3 minutes, or until it is well cooked completely, then drain and leave to cool. Peel the skin as well as any brown fat from the salmon once it has cooled. Chop the watercress and combine it with the lemon zest, yogurt, and half of the lemon juice to make the sauce. Warm the blinis for 1–2 minutes each side in a dry frying pan. Spread a little cream cheese over each blini and top with flaked salmon. Finish with a drizzle of the remaining lemon juice and blobs of the watercress sauce.

Nutritional Values: Calories: 63 kcal
/Carbohydrates: 3 g /Protein: 4 g /Fat: 4 g/Sodium: 180 mg

Scallops with Lime and Chilli Butter

Total Time: 20 mins / **Prep. Time:** 10 mins
/**Cooking Time:** 5 mins /**Difficulty:** Easy
/**Serving Size:** 4 servings

Ingredients:

- 1 tbsp. olive oil
- 2 tbsp. butter, softened
- 1 lime juice and grated rind
- 1 red chilli, finely chopped
- 12 scallops, cleaned
- ½ tsp. black pepper
- rocket leaves, to serve

Instructions:

In a small mixing bowl, combine the oil, butter, chilli, lime rind, and juice. Heat the butter mixture in a nonstick frying pan until it bubbles. Cook scallops for 1 minute on each side after adding them to the pan. Remove scallops from the pan and top with a sprig of rocket and a drizzle of pan juices.

Nutritional Values: Calories: 153 kcal
/Carbohydrates: 0.1 g /Protein: 21 g /Fat: 7 g/Sodium: 490 mg

Tiny Crab Tartlets

Total Time: 35 mins / **Prep. Time:** 20 mins
/**Cooking Time:** 15 mins /**Difficulty:** Easy
/**Serving Size:** 36 servings

Ingredients:

- 36 little pastry cases
- 4 tbsp. crème fraiche
- 1 egg, beaten
- pinch of paprika
- 1 tbsp. fresh chives, snipped
- 1 tbsp. Parmesan cheese, finely grated
- ¼ tsp. black pepper
- 225g fresh white crab meat

Instructions:

Preheat the oven to 450°F. On a baking sheet, place the pastry cases. Combine the remaining ingredients in a mixing bowl and use it to fill the pastry cases. Bake for 15 minutes, or until the filling is just firm and starting to turn brown. Allow to cool slightly before serving.

Nutritional Values: Calories: 22 kcal
/Carbohydrates: 1 g /Protein: 2 g /Fat: 1 g/Sodium: 130 mg

Chinese Steamed Trout

Total Time: 18 mins / **Prep. Time:** 10 mins
/**Cooking Time:** 8 mins /**Difficulty:** Easy
/**Serving Size:** 2 servings

Ingredients:

- 4 rainbow trout fillets, prepared
- 1 tbsp. low-sodium soy sauce
- 1 tbsp. sesame oil
- 1 lime grated rind and juice
- ¼ inch piece ginger, grated
- 2 cloves garlic, sliced
- 1 bunch spring onions, sliced

Instructions:

Place the fish on top of a piece of baking parchment in a big steamer. Combine the other ingredients in a bowl and pour over the fish. Steam for 6-8 minutes, or until the fish is done, covered with the lid. Serve with spaghetti, rice, or stir-fried vegetables.

Nutritional Values: Calories: 325 kcal /Carbohydrates: 4 g /Protein: 40 g /Fat: 16 g/Sodium: 110 mg

Fish Parcels

Total Time: 25 mins / **Prep. Time:** 10 mins /**Cooking Time:** 15 mins /**Difficulty:** Easy /**Serving Size:** 1 serving

Ingredients:

- 1 white fish fillet, skinned
- 215g can butter beans
- 1 large leek, finely sliced
- 1 tbsp. crème fraîche mixed
- sprig parsley, chopped
- ¼ tsp. black pepper
- Lemon slice for garnish

Instructions:

Preheat the oven to 450°F. Cut a huge piece of foil out of roll. Fill the foil with the leeks, fish, beans, and parsley, then spread over the crème fraîche, season it with pepper, then fold and fasten into a bundle. Place the parcel on baking sheet and bake for 15 minutes in a baking oven. Transfer the parcel to a serving platter after opening it. Serve with a slice of lemon.

Nutritional Values: Calories: 314 kcal /Carbohydrates: 23 g /Protein: 40 g /Fat: 5 g/Sodium: 500 mg

Prawn and Dill Open Sandwich

Total Time: 7 mins / **Prep. Time:** 5 mins /**Cooking Time:** 2 mins /**Difficulty:** Easy

Serving Size: 1 serving

Ingredients:

- 1 brown sandwich thin, halved
- 1 sprig fresh dill
- 80g cottage cheese, low-fat
- ¼ cucumber, thinly sliced
- 1 splash Tabasco sauce
- 5 cooked and peeled king prawns

Instructions:

Toast the thin sandwich halves lightly. Combine the snipped dill, cottage cheese, Tabasco, and black pepper in a mixing bowl. Spread the mixture evenly on top of the sandwich thins, then top with prawns, cucumber slices, extra dill, and serve.

Nutritional Values: Calories: 201 kcal /Carbohydrates: 22 g /Protein: 21 g /Fat: 3 g/Sodium: 170 mg

Trout with Basil and Citrus Sauce

Total Time: 20 mins / **Prep. Time:** 10 mins /**Cooking Time:** 10 mins /**Difficulty:** Easy /**Serving Size:** 2 servings

Ingredients:

- 2 boneless, skinless trout fillets
- 2 tbsp. fresh basil, torn
- 1 orange juice and zest
- ¼ tsp. black pepper
- 2 tbsp. low-fat cream

Instructions:

In a nonstick frying pan, place the fish fillets. Pour in the orange juice and zest, cover, and cook until the fish is done, about 5–6 minutes. Add the basil and cream to the fish and stir gently. Season the sauce with salt and pepper to taste. Serve and enjoy.

Nutritional Values: Calories: 166 kcal /Carbohydrates: 4 g /Protein: 20 g /Fat: 8 g/Sodium: 290 mg

Green Masala Fish Curry

Total Time: 27 mins / **Prep. Time:** 15 mins /**Cooking Time:** 12 mins /**Difficulty:** Medium /**Serving Size:** 2 servings

Ingredients:

- 75g fresh coriander, chopped
- 30g parsley, chopped
- 10g fresh mint, roughly chopped
- ¾ cup water
- 1 lime juice
- 2 tsp. rapeseed oil

- 1 red pepper, thinly sliced
- 1 onion, finely chopped
- ¼ inch ginger, finely chopped
- 1 chilli, finely chopped
- 2 tsp. mild curry powder
- 100g cod, large chunks
- 2 cloves garlic, crushed
- 100g salmon, large chunks

Instructions:

Blend the mint, coriander, lime juice, parsley, and water and form a paste. In a pan, heat the oil, and then add red pepper and onion. Cook the onions and pepper for 3–4 minutes, or until softened. Stir in the ginger, chilli, and garlic and cook for 1–2 minutes. Mix thoroughly for another minute after adding the curry powder. Place the fish in the pan and cover it in all of the spices, being careful not to break up the pieces of fish. Pour in the prepared green paste, bring to a mild boil, then reduce to a low heat and simmer for 3–4 minutes, turning periodically, until the fish is cooked through. Serve with lime wedges and coriander sprigs.

Nutritional Values: Calories: 259 kcal /Carbohydrates: 12 g /Protein: 22 g /Fat: 12 g/Sodium: 290 mg

Bagels with Smoked Salmon Spread

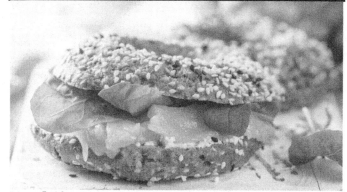

Total Time: 10 mins / **Prep. Time:** 10 mins /**Cooking Time:** N/A /**Difficulty:** Easy

Serving Size: 4 servings

Ingredients:

- 4 tbsp. low-fat soft cheese
- 4 mini bagels
- 2 tsp capers, roughly chopped
- ½ lemon juice and zest
- Few fresh chives, snipped

- ½ bunch fresh parsley, chopped
- 80g smoked salmon, chopped

Instructions:

Combine the lemon juice and zest, soft cheese, herbs, capers and salmon in a mixing bowl. Split the small bagels and toast them, then place the salmon mixture on top and serve.

Nutritional Values: Calories: 332 kcal /Carbohydrates: 46 g /Protein: 22 g /Fat: 6 g/Sodium: 240 mg

Asian Salmon Fillets

Total Time: 18 mins / **Prep. Time:** 10 mins /**Cooking Time:** 8 mins /**Difficulty:** Medium /**Serving Size:** 6 servings

Ingredients:

- 6 pieces salmon fillet
- 2 tsp. sesame oil
- 1 tbsp. low-salt soy sauce
- 1 tsp. fresh ginger, grated
- pinch of chilli flakes
- Fresh coriander, for garnish
- 2 tsp. runny honey
- 4 spring onions, shredded
- Spring onions, for garnish

Instructions:

In a non-metallic bowl, combine all of the marinade ingredients except fish and whisk thoroughly. Add the salmon fillets, toss them in the marinade, and leave them aside to absorb the flavors. Cook for 3–4 minutes over medium heat, then flip over and cook for another 3–4 minutes on the other side. Before serving, garnish with coriander and spring onions.

Nutritional Values: Calories: 293 kcal /Carbohydrates: 3 g /Protein: 26 g /Fat: 20 g/Sodium: 400 mg

Crab Cakes

Total Time: 25 mins / **Prep. Time:** 15 mins /**Cooking Time:** 10 mins /**Difficulty:** Easy /**Serving Size:** 8 servings

Ingredients:

- 1 lb. lump crab meat
- 2 eggs, slightly beaten
- 1½ cups bread crumbs
- 2 scallions, thinly sliced
- ½ red bell pepper, finely chopped

- 1 tsp. Old Bay seasoning
- ¼ tsp. cayenne pepper
- 1 tbsp. fat-free mayonnaise
- 2 tsp. canola oil

Instructions:

Combine the bread crumbs, crab, bell pepper, eggs, mayonnaise, scallions, cayenne pepper and Old Bay seasoning in a medium mixing bowl and mix well. Form the batter into eight circular cakes. Heat the oil in a large pan over medium heat. Cook the crab cakes for 8 to 10 minutes, or till golden brown, flipping once in a while.

Nutritional Values: Calories: 106 kcal /Carbohydrates: 5.4 g /Protein: 13 g /Fat: 3 g/Sodium: 387 mg

Lemon Scallops

Total Time: 25 mins / **Prep. Time:** 15 mins /**Cooking Time:** 10 mins /**Difficulty:** Medium/**Serving Size:** 4 servings

Ingredients:

- ¼ tsp. black pepper
- 1 lb. sea scallops, patted dry
- 1 egg
- 1 tsp. onion powder
- Paprika, for garnish
- ¼ cup Italian-flavored bread crumbs
- 1 tbsp. water
- Cooking spray
- 1 tbsp. lemon juice

Instructions:

Preheat the oven to 450°F. Use a cooking spray to coat a rimmed baking sheet. Scallops should be seasoned with onion powder and black pepper. Whisk together the egg and water in a small bowl. In a separate shallow dish, place the bread crumbs. Cover each marinated scallop in the egg mixture, then gently coat in bread crumbs. Place the scallops on the baking sheet, gently spraying the tops with cooking spray and, if preferred, paprika. Bake for 10 to 12 minutes in the oven, or until golden and firm in the centre. Serve right away with a squeeze of lemon juice.

Nutritional Values: Calories: 126 kcal /Carbohydrates: 10 g /Protein: 16 g /Fat: 2 g/Sodium: 593 mg

Chapter 14: Meat Recipes

When you're diagnosed with diabetes, it doesn't always mean you have to stop eating meat. However, it does suggest that you should be a little more selective about the meat you eat.

Lean meat, fish, shellfish, and poultry are suitable for diabetics. To lower the risk of high cholesterol and heart disease, they should avoid Tran's fats or meats high in saturated fats.

In this chapter, you'll find several delicious and healthy meat recipes for diabetics.

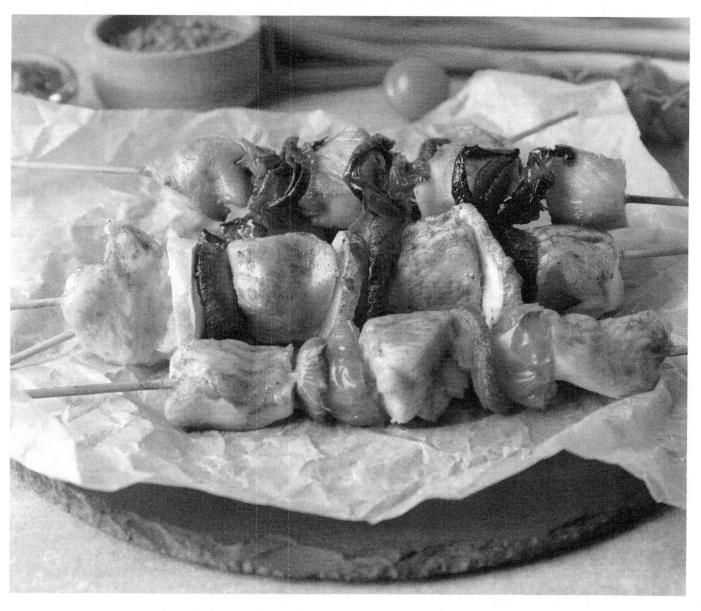

Mediterranean Pork Chops

Total Time: 45 mins / **Prep. Time:** 10 mins /**Cooking Time:** 35 mins /**Difficulty:** Medium /**Serving Size:** 4 servings

Ingredients:

- 4 boneless pork loin chops
- ¼ tsp. black pepper
- ¼ tsp. salt
- 3 cloves garlic, minced
- 1 tbsp. fresh rosemary, finely snipped

Instructions:

Preheat the oven to 425°F. Wrap a shallow roasting pan using aluminium foil. Season the chops on all sides with salt and pepper and put aside. Combine garlic and rosemary in a small bowl. Apply the rosemary mixture to all sides of the chops and massage it in with your fingertips. In the prepared roasting pan, arrange the chops on a rack. Chops should be roasted for 10 minutes. Reduce the oven temperature to 350°F and continue roasting for another 25 minutes, or until no pink remains and the juices flow clear.

Nutritional Values: Calories: 161 kcal /Carbohydrates: 1 g /Protein: 25 g /Fat: 5 g/Sodium: 192 mg

Lamb Chops

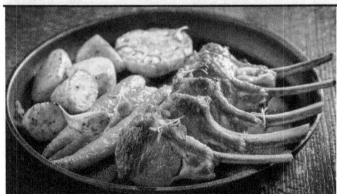

Total Time: 40 mins / **Prep. Time:** 30 mins /**Cooking Time:** 10 mins /**Difficulty:** Medium/**Serving Size:** 4 servings

Ingredients:

- ¼ cup olive oil
- 1 tbsp. fresh rosemary, chopped
- 2 tbsp. red-wine vinegar

- 1 tsp. grated lemon zest
- 1½ tsp. fresh oregano, chopped
- ¾ tsp. cracked black pepper
- 1 clove garlic, grated
- 8 lamb chops
- ½ tsp. salt

Instructions:

In a large zip-top plastic bag, combine the vinegar, oil, oregano, rosemary, garlic, lemon zest, and pepper. Salt the chops and set them in the bag. Rub the prepared marinade into the chops and set aside for 20 minutes at room temperature, rotating periodically. Preheat the air fryer to 380°F. Coat the basket with cooking spray and put the chops in a single layer in it. Cook the chops for about 4 minutes, or until the chops are gently browned. Cook the chops for next 4 to 5 minutes on the other side, or until medium-rare.

Nutritional Values: Calories: 133 kcal /Carbohydrates: 4 g /Protein: 16 g /Fat: 7 g/Sodium: 336 mg

Mediterranean Meatballs

Total Time: 30 mins / **Prep. Time:** 10 mins /**Cooking Time:** 30 mins /**Difficulty:** Easy /**Serving Size:** 8 servings

Ingredients:

- 12 oz. roasted red peppers
- 2 eggs lightly beaten
- 1½ cups whole-wheat bread crumbs
- ½ cup fresh basil, snipped
- 1/3 cup tomato sauce
- ½ tsp. salt
- ¼ tsp. ground black pepper
- ¼ cup fresh flat-leaf parsley, snipped
- 2 lb. lean ground beef

Instructions:

Combine bread crumbs, roasted red peppers, beaten eggs, basil, tomato sauce, parsley, salt, and pepper in a large mixing bowl. Mix in the ground beef well. Make 48 meatballs out of the meat mixture. Place meatballs in a 15x10x1-inch baking tray lined with foil. Preheat oven to 350°F and bake for 20 minutes, or until done.

Nutritional Values: Calories: 94 kcal /Carbohydrates: 2.5 g /Protein: 13 g /Fat: 3 g/Sodium: 170 mg

Garlic Beef

Total Time: 25 mins / **Prep. Time:** 10 mins /**Cooking Time:** 15 mins /**Difficulty:** Easy /**Serving Size:** 4 servings

Ingredients:

- 1 tsp. sesame oil
- 10 oz. frozen chopped broccoli
- 1 lb. beef eye of round, thin strips
- 1 tbsp. light soy sauce
- 1 tbsp. minced garlic
- ¼ tsp. black pepper

Instructions:

In a 12-inch nonstick skillet, heat the oil over high heat. Combine the beef, garlic, broccoli, soy sauce, and pepper in a large mixing bowl. Cook it for 15 minutes, stirring periodically, or until meat is tender.

Nutritional Values: Calories: 214 kcal /Carbohydrates: 6 g /Protein: 27 g /Fat: 9 g/Sodium: 320 mg

Balsamic Beef, Onions, and Mushrooms

Total Time: 35 mins / **Prep. Time:** 10 mins /**Cooking Time:** 25 mins /**Difficulty:** Medium /**Serving Size:** 4 servings

Ingredients:

- 2 large sweet onions, sliced
- ½ tsp. salt, divided
- 3 tsp. olive oil, divided
- 1 cup mushrooms, sliced
- 5 tsp. balsamic vinegar, divided
- ¼ tsp. dried thyme
- 1 lb. beef top sirloin, ½ inch-thick slices
- ½ tsp. black pepper

Instructions:

Over medium heat, heat a large nonstick skillet. Add 2 tsp. olive oil and onions. Cook and stir for 15 minutes after adding the onions. Whisk together 3 tsp. balsamic vinegar with 1/4 tsp. salt. Add 1 tsp. at a time, scraping out browned pieces with a spatula. Reduce the heat to a medium-low setting and add mushrooms in the pan. Cook, stirring occasionally, for 4 to 5 minutes, or until mushrooms are soft. Place in a medium mixing dish. Set aside, covered. Raise the temperature to medium-high. Add beef in the pan with remaining 1 tsp. oil. Sprinkle the remaining 1/4

tsp. salt, pepper and thyme over the meat. Cook for 4–6 minutes, or until golden brown. Turn the heat off. Over the steak, drizzle the remaining 2 tsp. balsamic vinegar. Toss in the vegetables. Serve right away.

Nutritional Values: Calories: 216 kcal /Carbohydrates: 7 g /Protein: 26 g /Fat: 9 g/Sodium: 360 mg

Orange-Pomegranate Glazed Ham

Total Time: 2 hours 30 mins / **Prep. Time:** 30 mins /**Cooking Time:** 2 hours /**Difficulty:** Medium/**Serving Size:** 36 servings

Ingredients:

- 9 lbs. spiral-cut smoked ham half
- 3 tbsp. orange marmalade
- 1 cup pomegranate juice
- ½ tsp. Dijon mustard
- ¼ tsp. ground cloves

Instructions:

Preheat the oven to 350°F. Trim the fat from the ham once it has been unwrapped. Place on roasting pan, flat side down. Cover with foil, but only loosely. Bake for 1 hour and 45 minutes in the oven. Meanwhile, in a small saucepan over medium heat, warm the juice. Reduce heat to medium-low and continue to simmer for another 40 minutes or until the juice has been reduced to approximately 1/4 cup. Turn off the heat in the pan. Allow for a 10-minute cooling period. Stir in the cloves, marmalade, and mustard until thoroughly combined. Remove the foil from the ham and coat it with the orange-pomegranate glaze evenly. Bake for another 15 minutes in the oven Allow for 5 minutes of resting time before slicing and serving.

Nutritional Values: Calories: 122 kcal /Carbohydrates: 5 g /Protein: 11 g /Fat: 7 g/Sodium: 794 mg

Roasted Pork

Total Time: 40 mins / **Prep. Time:** 10 mins /**Cooking Time:** 30 mins /**Difficulty:** Medium /**Serving Size:** 4 servings

Ingredients:

- 3 tbsp. barbecue sauce
- 1 tbsp. dry sherry

- 1 tbsp. low-sodium soy sauce
- ½ tsp. crushed peppercorns
- 2 cloves garlic, minced
- 2 whole pork tenderloins

Instructions:

Preheat the oven to 350°F. In a small bowl, combine the soy sauce, garlic, barbecue sauce, sherry, and peppercorns. One-fourth of the mixture should be applied equally to each side of roast. Place the roasts on a rack in a shallow roasting pan coated with foil. Cook for 15 minutes on one side, then flip and brush with the remaining barbecue sauce mixture. Cook until an internal temperature of 165°F is reached. It will take around 30 minutes. Place the roast on a chopping board and cover it with foil. Allow 10 to 15 minutes to rest before cutting. During this time, the inside temperature will rise by 5 to 10 degrees Fahrenheit. If preferred, slice diagonally and serve warm with rice. Cut into parts and store in the refrigerator for up to 3 days or freeze for up to 3 months for use in other recipes.

Nutritional Values: Calories: 199 kcal /Carbohydrates: 3 g /Protein: 32 g /Fat: 5 g/Sodium: 301 mg

Oven-Fried Pork Chops

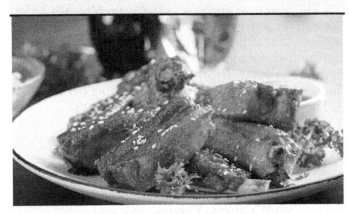

Total Time: 35 mins / **Prep. Time:** 15 mins /**Cooking Time:** 20 mins /**Difficulty:** Easy /**Serving Size:** 4 servings

Ingredients:

- Cooking spray
- 1 large egg, lightly beaten
- ¼ cup all-purpose flour
- ¾ cup whole-wheat breadcrumbs
- 1 tsp. Dijon mustard
- ½ tsp. kosher salt
- 1 tsp. ground pepper

- 4 boneless pork chops

Instructions:

Preheat oven to 400°F. Coat a wire rack with cooking spray and place it on a large baking sheet. Fill a small dish halfway with flour. In a separate small bowl, whisk together the beaten egg and mustard. In a third shallow dish, combine panko and pepper. Season the pork on both sides with salt. Using flour, dredge each pork chop and shake off the excess. Coat the pork in the egg mixture, then in the panko, pressing firmly to adhere. Place on the rack that has been prepared. Using frying spray, coat the pork chops. Bake for 18 to 20 minutes, or until the chops are golden brown and cooked through.

Nutritional Values: Calories: 194 kcal /Carbohydrates: 11 g /Protein: 21 g /Fat: 6 g/Sodium: 325 mg

Mushroom-Sauced Pork Chops

Total Time: 4 hour 30 0 mins / **Prep. Time:** 30 mins /**Cooking Time:** 4 hours /**Difficulty:** Easy /**Serving Size:** 6 servings

Ingredients:

- 4 pork loin chops
- 1 small onion, thinly sliced
- 1 tbsp. cooking oil
- 6 Fresh thyme sprigs
- 10 oz. low-fat cream of mushroom soup
- ½ cup apple juice, no sugar
- 2 tbsp. quick-cooking tapioca
- 2 tsp. fresh thyme, snipped
- ¼ tsp. garlic powder
- 1½ tsp. Worcestershire sauce
- 1½ cups sliced fresh mushrooms

Instructions:

Chops should be fat-free. Heat the oil in a large skillet over medium heat. Cook until chops are browned, rotating to ensure even browning. Remove any excess fat. In a 3-1/2- or 4-quart slow cooker, place the onion. Toss in the chops. Crush the tapioca with a mortar and pestle. Combine the tapioca, apple juice, mushroom soup, snipped thyme, Worcestershire sauce, and garlic powder in a medium mixing bowl; whisk in the mushrooms. Pour the sauce over the chops in the slow cooker. Cover and cook on high for 4 to 4-1/2 hours. Garnish with thyme sprigs and serve.

Nutritional Values: Calories: 220 kcal /Carbohydrates: 11 g /Protein: 26 g /Fat: 6 g/Sodium: 233 mg

Mediterranean Brisket

Total Time: 5 hour 25 mins / **Prep. Time:** 25 mins /**Cooking Time:** 5 hours /**Difficulty:** Medium/**Serving Size:** 6 servings

Ingredients:

- 3 lb. fresh beef brisket
- 2 medium fennel bulbs, wedges
- 3 tsp. dried Italian seasoning, crushed
- ½ cup beef broth, lower sodium
- 14 oz. can dice tomatoes, no-salt-added
- 1 tsp. lemon peel, finely shredded
- ½ cup pitted olives
- ¼ tsp. ground black pepper
- ¼ tsp. salt
- 2 tbsp. all-purpose flour
- ¼ cup cold water
- 1 cup Fresh parsley

Instructions:

Trim any excess fat from the meat. 1 teaspoon Italian spice should be sprinkled on the meat. Place the meat in a slow cooker with a capacity of 3 1/2 to 4 quarts. Fennel should be sprinkled on top. Toss tomatoes, olives, broth, salt, lemon peel, pepper, and the remainder 2 teaspoons Italian seasoning together. Pour everything into the cooker. Cook on high heat for 5 hours, covered. Remove the meat from the cooker and set aside the juices. Meat should be sliced. Arrange the meat and veggies on a dish and keep them warm by covering them. Skim the fat from the juices and pour them into a glass measuring cup. Measure 2 cups of the liquids for the sauce. Place in a saucepan. Combine the flour and cold water in a small basin; stir into the pot. Cook, stirring constantly, until the sauce has thickened and is bubbling. Serve the sauce beside the meat. Garnish with parsley and more lemon peel if desired.

Nutritional Values: Calories: 254 kcal /Carbohydrates: 10 g /Protein: 34 g /Fat: 8 g/Sodium: 336 mg

Asian Beef Kabobs

Total Time: 22 mins / **Prep. Time:** 10 mins /**Cooking Time:** 12 mins /**Difficulty:** Easy /**Serving Size:** 8 servings

Ingredients:

- 1 lb. beef Sirloin Steak Boneless, cubes
- 2 tbsp. dry sherry
- ¼ cup hoisin sauce
- 1 tsp. dark sesame oil
- 2 tsp. packed light brown sugar
- 6 green onions, sliced diagonally

Instructions:

Whisk together the hoisin sauce, brown sugar, sherry and sesame oil. Trim any excess fat from the beef steak. Cut the meat into 1/4-inch-thick pieces crosswise. Thread meat and green onion slices onto skewers alternately, weaving back and forth. Place the kabobs on the rack in the broiler pan, 3 to 4 inches away from the heat. Half of the hoisin mixture should be brushed on. Broil for 9 to 12 minutes, flipping once and sprinkling with the remaining hoisin mixture before serving.

Nutritional Values: Calories: 53 kcal /Carbohydrates: 2 g /Protein: 7 g /Fat: 2 g/Sodium: 47 mg

Swedish Meatballs

Total Time: 30 mins / **Prep. Time:** 10 mins /**Cooking Time:** 20 mins /**Difficulty:** Medium/**Serving Size:** 32 servings

Ingredients:

- 1 lb. Lean Ground Beef
- 4 tsp. dried dill
- 1 egg
- 2 tbsp. fine, plain breadcrumbs
- 2 onions, finely chopped
- 1 tbsp. butter
- 4 tsp. allspice
- 1 cup beef stock
- 1 tbsp. flour
- 1 tbsp. sour cream
- 1 cup skim milk
- 4 tsp. black pepper

Instructions:

Preheat the oven to 350°F. Combine beef, 1 teaspoon dill, breadcrumbs, onion, egg, and allspice in a mixing bowl. Mix thoroughly. Form 1 tablespoon meatballs out of the mixture. Arrange meatballs on broiling tray and bake for 10 minutes, or until meatballs are no longer pink. Heat the butter in a skillet over medium high heat while the meatballs are baking. Cook stirring frequently, for about 4 minutes after whisking in the flour. Slowly whisk in the beef stock, whisking constantly over low heat until no lumps remain. Continue whisking while carefully adding skim milk, stirring constantly until no lumps remain. Reduce the heat to low and simmer for 5 minutes, stirring often. Remove the pan from the heat. Combine the remaining dill, sour cream, and black pepper in a mixing bowl. When the meatballs are done, add them to the sauce in the pan, heat through, and serve right away.

Nutritional Values: Calories: 170 kcal /Carbohydrates: 14 g /Protein: 12 g /Fat: 8 g/Sodium: 141 mg

Pepper Beef Steak

Total Time: 41 mins / **Prep. Time:** 30 mins /**Cooking Time:** 11 mins /**Difficulty:** Medium/**Serving Size:** 4 servings

Ingredients:

- 1/3 cup Dijon-style mustard
- 4 beef steaks, cut 3/4 inch thick
- 2 tsp. ground cumin
- 2 tbsp. mixed peppercorns, coarsely ground
- 1 tsp. garlic, minced
- ¼ cup butter, softened
- 1 tbsp. fresh cilantro, minced
- 2 mild green chili peppers

Instructions:

In a small bowl, combine peppercorns, mustard, and cumin. Remove half and set aside for brushing. The leftover mustard mixture should be spread on both sides of the steaks. Refrigerate for 30 minutes after covering. In a small bowl, combine the cilantro, butter, and garlic. Over medium, ash-covered coals, place steaks and peppers on the grid. Grill, covered, for 11 minutes until steaks are medium rare and peppers are blackened, rotating periodically, and brushing steaks with conserved mustard mixture during the final 4 minutes. Remove the charred peppers from the pan, cover, and set aside for 5 minutes. Skin, stems, and seeds should all be removed. Chop the peppers and add half of them to the butter mixture. Pour 1 teaspoon butter mixture on top of each steak Add the remaining chopped peppers on top. With the remaining butter, serve.

Nutritional Values: Calories: 278 kcal

/Carbohydrates: 9 g /Protein: 37 g /Fat: 1 g/Sodium: 580 mg

Mediterranean Braised Beef

Total Time: 2 hour 15 mins / **Prep. Time:** 15 mins /**Cooking Time:** 2 hours /**Difficulty:** Medium/**Serving Size:** 6 servings

Ingredients:

- 3 lb. beef chuck shoulder pot roast, boneless
- 2 tbsp. olive oil
- ¼ cup all-purpose flour
- 2 small onions, sliced
- ½ tsp. salt
- ¼ cup balsamic vinegar
- ¼ cup chopped pitted dates
- 4 medium shallots, sliced
- ½ tsp. black pepper

Instructions:

Preheat the oven to 325°F. Using flour, lightly coat the beef pot roast. In a Dutch oven, heat the oil over medium heat until it is hot. Remove the pot roast when it has been browned. In a Dutch oven, combine 1-1/2 cups water and vinegar; simmer and stir until brown pieces stuck to the pan are dissolved. Return the pot roast to the oven. Bring to a boil with the onions, shallots, dates, salt, and pepper. Cook in a 325°F oven for 2 hours. Remove the pot roast from the oven and keep it warm. Cook liquid and veggies to desired consistency over medium-high heat. Carve up the pot roast. Serve with a side of sauce.

Nutritional Values: Calories: 290 kcal /Carbohydrates: 16 g /Protein: 29 g /Fat: 12 g/Sodium: 275 mg

Speedy Steak

Total Time: 18 mins / **Prep. Time:** 10 mins /**Cooking Time:** 8 mins /**Difficulty:** Easy /**Serving Size:** 6 servings

Ingredients:

- 1 tbsp. canola oil
- 2 garlic cloves, minced
- 3 cups mix vegetables, sliced
- 2 tbsp. lite soy sauce
- 1½ lb. lean sirloin steak, cooked and sliced
- 1 tbsp. dry sherry
- 2 tbsp. brown sugar

- 2 tbsp. sesame seeds, toasted
- 3 cups cooked rice

Instructions:

In a wok, heat the oil over high heat. Stir-fry the veggies for 4 minutes. Stir in the garlic and cook for another 2 minutes. Stir in the beef and after 1 minute add the sugar, soy sauce, and sherry to the pan and stir to combine. Cover with a napkin and steam for 1 minute. Serve with sesame seeds on top of rice.

Nutritional Values: Calories: 303 kcal /Carbohydrates: 33 g /Protein: 28 g /Fat: 6 g/Sodium: 282 mg

Pepper Steak with Mustard Sauce

Total Time: 25 mins / **Prep. Time:** 10 mins /**Cooking Time:** 15 mins /**Difficulty:** Easy /**Serving Size:** 4 servings

Ingredients:

- 4 beef tenderloin steaks
- cooking spray
- 2 tsp. coarsely ground black pepper
- 1/3 cup dry red wine
- 2 garlic cloves, minced
- 1 tbsp. Dijon mustard
- 1/3 cup low-salt beef broth

Instructions:

Season the steaks on both sides with pepper. O a medium nonstick skillet sprayed with cooking spray over medium heat. Place the steaks in a single layer in the pan and sear for about 1 minute, or until browned. Cook for another 8 minutes, or until desired doneness is reached, flipping once. If there is any liquid fat in the pan, drain it. Cook, stirring constantly, for 1 minute or until light brown. Boil for 1 minute after adding the wine and broth. Remove the steaks from the skillet and keep them warm by covering them. Stir in the mustard with a wire whisk until the sauce is fully combined. Serve the sauce on top of the steaks.

Nutritional Values: Calories: 207 kcal /Carbohydrates: 0 g /Protein: 23 g /Fat: 9 g/Sodium: 92 mg

Mustard Roast Beef

Total Time: 50 mins / **Prep. Time:** 10 mins /**Cooking Time:** 40 mins /**Difficulty:** Easy

/Serving Size: 8 servings

Ingredients:

- ¼ cup apricot preserves
- 1 tbsp. light brown sugar
- 2 tbsp. spicy brown mustard
- 3 tsp. reduced-sodium Worcestershire sauce
- 1 tsp. caraway seeds, crushed
- 1 tbsp. prepared horseradish
- 1 tsp. crushed black peppercorns
- ¼ tsp. ground allspice
- 2 lb. boneless beef sirloin tip roast, fat trimmed

Instructions:

In a medium mixing dish, combine all ingredients except the beef. Apply to all of the meat's surfaces. In a roasting pan, place the meat on a rack. Roast for 40 minutes at 350°F. Serve and enjoy.

Nutritional Values: Calories: 171 kcal /Carbohydrates: 9 g /Protein: 20 g /Fat: 5 g/Sodium: 118 mg

Rosemary-Sage Steak

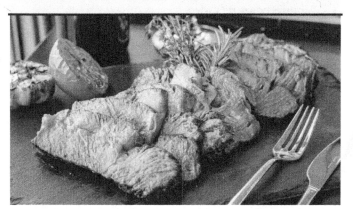

Total Time: 1 hour 25 mins / **Prep. Time:** 1 hour mins /**Cooking Time:** 25 mins /**Difficulty:** Medium/**Serving Size:** 8 servings

Ingredients:

- 2 lb. boneless top sirloin steak
- ¼ cup fresh lemon juice
- 3 tbsp. dry white wine
- ½ cup chopped onion
- 2 tbsp. sage, finely chopped
- 2 tbsp. fresh rosemary, finely chopped
- 3 cloves garlic, minced
- 1 tbsp. Dijon mustard
- ½ tsp. pepper
- 1 tsp. olive oil
- ¼ tsp. salt

Instructions:

Place the steak in a plastic bag that is airtight. Combine all the ingredients in a small bowl. Pour the sauce over the meat and flip it to coat it evenly. Refrigerate for 1 hour rotating once or twice. Preheat the grill to medium-high. Drain the steak and grill it for 8 to 12 minutes each side, or until done to your liking.

Nutritional Values: Calories: 116 kcal /Carbohydrates: 0 g /Protein: 25 g /Fat: 6 g/Sodium: 150 mg

Salmon with Peanut Butter Sauce

Total Time: 30 mins / **Prep. Time:** 10 mins /**Cooking Time:** 20 mins /**Difficulty:** Easy /**Serving Size:** 4 servings

Ingredients:

- 1 lb. salmon
- 2 tsp. chili garlic sauce
- freshly ground pepper, to taste
- ¼ cup peanut butter
- 1 tsp. olive oil
- ¼ cup orange juice

Instructions:

Preheat the oven to 400°F and line a baking sheet with aluminum foil. Place the salmon on a baking sheet, sprinkle with olive oil, and season to taste with pepper. Bake it for 15-20 minutes, or until salmon is cooked through. Whisk together peanut butter, chili garlic sauce, and orange juice in a small sauce pot over medium-low heat until heated. Pour the peanut butter sauce over the fish to serve.

Nutritional Values: Calories: 334 kcal /Carbohydrates: 5 g /Protein: 27 g /Fat: 23 g/Sodium: 173 mg

Montreal-Style Salmon

Total Time: 15 mins / **Prep. Time:** 5 mins /**Cooking Time:** 10 mins /**Difficulty:** Easy /**Serving Size:** 2 servings

Ingredients:

- ½ lb. salmon fillets
- ½ tsp. Steak Seasoning
- 1/8 tsp. Dill Weed
- ½ tsp. grated lemon peel

Instructions:

In a small bowl, combine Steak Seasoning, lemon peel, and dill weed. Rub the mixture all over the fish. Allow for a 5-minute rest period. Grill salmon, skin side down, for 10 to 12 minutes over medium heat, or until it flakes easily with a fork.

Nutritional Values: Calories: 168 kcal /Carbohydrates: 0 g /Protein: 24 g /Fat: 8 g/Sodium: 174 mg

Chapter 15: Snack Recipes

Snacks are smaller foods that are consumed in between meals. People having type-2 diabetes should consume snacks that are high in fiber, protein, and healthy fats, since they help you to maintain energy for long time period. Snacks can help you lose weight by controlling appetite and keeping you full between meals if you plan and focus on nutrient-dense foods.

In this chapter, you'll find several healthy and delicious snacks recipe for people with type-2 diabetes.

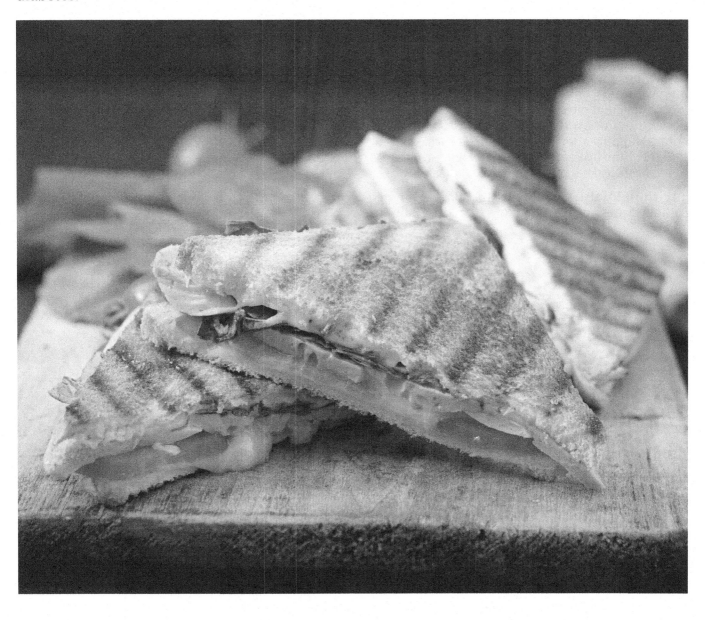

Baked Turnip Fries

Total Time: 40 mins / **Prep. Time:** 10 mins /**Cooking Time:** 30 mins /**Difficulty:** Easy /**Serving Size:** 1 serving

Ingredients:

- ¼ tsp. garlic powder
- ¼ tsp. paprika
- ¼ tsp. onion powder
- 1 turnip
- ¼ tsp. salt
- 1 tbsp. olive oil

Instructions:

Preheat the oven to 425°F. Turnips should be peeled and chopped into strips like fries. In a mixing bowl, combine turnips, onion powder, paprika, garlic powder, salt, and olive oil. Lay out fries evenly on a baking sheet lined with foil. Bake the fries for 20 minutes, flipping after 10 minutes to ensure equal baking. For the last 2 minutes of cooking, turn the oven to broil. Take it out of the oven and eat it!

Nutritional Values: Calories: 50 kcal /Carbohydrates: 2 g /Protein: 0 g /Fat: 5 g/Sodium: 586 mg

Roasted Edamame

Total Time: 30 mins / **Prep. Time:** 5 mins /**Cooking Time:** 25 mins /**Difficulty:** Medium /**Serving Size:** 6 servings

Ingredients:

- 20 oz. frozen edamame, shelled
- 2 tbsp. balsamic vinegar
- 1 tsp. ground black pepper
- 1 tbsp. extra virgin olive oil
- sea salt to taste

Instructions:

Preheat the oven to 370°F. In a mixing bowl, combine frozen edamame with the balsamic vinegar, olive oil, sea salt and black pepper. Toss until they are evenly coated. Place the coated shells on a baking sheet in an equal layer and bake for 20 minutes. Set a 10-minute timer. Stir the mixture after 10 minutes. Return the edamame to the oven and cook for another 10 minutes, or until the edges are golden. Remove the dish from the oven. Serve on a platter or in a dish, and then eat the beans right out of the shell.

Nutritional Values: Calories: 81 kcal

/Carbohydrates: 4 g /Protein: 6 g /Fat: 4 g/Sodium: 4 mg

Crunchy Bean Snack

Total Time: 1 hour 5 mins / **Prep. Time:** 5 mins /**Cooking Time:** 60 mins/ **Difficulty:** Medium/**Serving Size:** 3 servings

Ingredients:

- 1 ½ cup garbanzo beans
- ½ tsp. cumin
- 1 tsp. olive oil
- pinch of salt

Instructions:

Preheat the oven to 300°F. In a small mixing dish, combine all of the ingredients. Garbanzo beans should be uniformly distributed on a baking sheet. Bake the beans in oven for 1 hour at 300 degrees. Stir the beans after every 15 minutes. Enjoy.

Nutritional Values: Calories: 157 kcal /Carbohydrates: 27 g /Protein: 6 g /Fat: 3 g/Sodium: 411 mg

Tuna Cucumber Bites

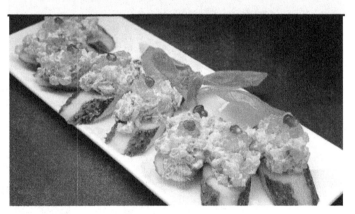

Total Time: 5 mins / **Prep. Time:** 5 mins /**Cooking Time:** N/A /**Difficulty:** Easy

Serving Size: 5 servings

Ingredients:

- 3 ½ oz. canned tuna
- ½ green onion chopped
- ½ tbsp. relish
- 1 tbsp. chopped onion
- ¾ cucumber

Instructions:

Slice cucumber into slices on a chopping board. There should be about 20 slices in all. To create the tuna salad, mix together tuna, relish, onion, mayo. Spread 1 tsp. tuna mix on top of each cucumber slice

Nutritional Values: Calories: 49 kcal /Carbohydrates: 2 g /Protein: 5 g /Fat: 2 g/Sodium: 81 mg

Broccoli-Cheddar Quinoa Bites

Total Time: 1 hour 5 mins / **Prep. Time:** 40 mins /**Cooking Time:** 25 mins /**Difficulty:** Medium/**Serving Size:** 8 servings

Ingredients:

- ½ cup quinoa
- ¾ cup broccoli, finely chopped
- ⅛ tsp. + ¼ tsp. salt, divided
- ½ tsp. baking powder
- ¾ cup Cheddar cheese shredded
- ¼ tsp. onion powder
- ½ tsp. garlic powder
- ¼ tsp. ground pepper
- Cooking spray
- 1 large egg, lightly beaten

Instructions:

Preheat the oven to 350°F. Use paper liners to line 16 cups of mini muffin tray or spray the pan with cooking spray. Cook quinoa according to package guidelines with 1/8 tsp. salt. Remove from heat and let aside for 5 minutes, covered. Allow it cool for at least 10 minutes in a large mixing dish. Toss the quinoa with the Cheddar, broccoli, garlic powder, baking powder, pepper, onion powder, and the remaining 1/4 tsp. salt. Add the egg and mix well. Using lightly wet fingertips push the quinoa mixture firmly into the prepared muffin cups. Use cooking spray to mist the tops of muffins. Bake for 22 to 25 minutes, or until brown. Allow to cool for 20 minutes in the pan on a wire rack before removing to the rack to cool fully.

Nutritional Values: Calories: 87 kcal /Carbohydrates: 8 g /Protein: 5 g /Fat: 4 g/Sodium: 209 mg

Roasted Buffalo Chickpeas

Total Time: 45 mins / **Prep. Time:** 10 mins /**Cooking Time:** 35 mins /**Difficulty:** Easy /**Serving Size:** 4 servings

Ingredients:

- 1 tbsp. white vinegar
- ¼ tsp. salt
- ½ tsp. cayenne pepper
- 15 oz. unsalted chickpeas, rinsed

Instructions:

Preheat oven to 400°F and place rack in upper third. In a large mixing dish, combine the cayenne, vinegar, and salt. Toss the chickpeas with the vinegar mixture after fully drying them. Place on a lined baking sheet to cool. Roast the chickpeas for 30 to 35 minutes, turning twice, until golden and crispy. Allow it cool for 30 minutes on the pan; the chickpeas will become crispy as they cool.

Nutritional Values: Calories: 109 kcal /Carbohydrates: 18 g /Protein: 6 g /Fat: 1 g/Sodium: 162 mg

Super-Seed Snack Bars

Total Time: 1 hour 5 mins / **Prep. Time:** 25 mins /**Cooking Time:** 35-40 mins /**Difficulty:** Medium /**Serving Size:** 25 servings

Ingredients:

- 1/3 cup tahini
- 1 tsp. vanilla extract
- 1/3 cup honey
- 1 cup unsweetened coconut, shredded
- ½ cup raw pepitas, unsalted
- ¼ cup chia seeds
- ½ cup sunflower seeds, unsalted
- ¼ cup hemp seeds
- ¼ tsp. salt

Instructions:

Preheat the oven to 325°F. Line an 8-inch-square baking sheet with parchment paper, keeping excess hanging over two edges. Use cooking spray to coat the parchment and sides of the pan. In a small saucepan, combine tahini and honey over medium heat. Cook stirring constantly, for approximately 2 minutes, or until well combined and warmed. Remove the pan from the heat and mix in the vanilla and salt. In a large mixing dish, combine pepitas, coconut, chia seeds, sunflower seeds, and hemp seeds. Stir in the tahini mixture until everything is uniformly covered. In the prepared pan, press the ingredients firmly. Bake for 30 to 35 minutes, or until brown. Allow to cool fully on a wire rack in the pan. Lift the uncut squares out with the overhanging parchment. Cut into 25 squares using a sharp knife. Serve and enjoy.

Nutritional Values: Calories: 110 kcal /Carbohydrates: 7 g /Protein: 3 g /Fat: 8 g/Sodium:

27 mg

Cranberry and Almond Granola Bars

Total Time: 1 hour 20 mins / **Prep. Time:** 10 mins /**Cooking Time:** 30 mins /**Difficulty:** Medium/**Serving Size:** 24 servings

Ingredients:

- 3 cups rolled oats
- 1 cup dried cranberries
- 1 cup crispy brown rice cereal
- ½ cup pecans, chopped
- ½ cup almonds, chopped
- ¼ tsp. salt
- ½ cup almond butter
- 2/3 cup brown rice syrup
- 1 tsp. vanilla extract

Instructions:

Preheat the oven to 325°F. Using parchment paper, line a 9*13-inch baking sheet, with excess parchment draping over two edges. Spray the parchment lightly with cooking spray. In a large mixing bowl, combine the rice cereal, oats, almonds, cranberries, pecans, and salt. In a microwave-safe bowl, combine almond butter, rice syrup, and vanilla and heat 30 seconds in the microwave. Stir in the wet ingredients into dry ingredients until everything is well mixed. Transfer to the prepared pan and use the back of a spatula to firmly press the dough into the pan. Bake for 20 to 25 minutes, or until just starting to brown around the edges but still soft in the centre, for chewier bars. Bake for 30 to 35 minutes, or until golden brown around the edges and somewhat hard in the centre, for crunchier bars. Cut into 24 bars, then set aside for another 30 minutes to cool fully without splitting the bars.

Nutritional Values: Calories: 161 kcal /Carbohydrates: 23 g /Protein: 3 g /Fat: 0.7 g/Sodium: 52 mg

Soy and Lime Roasted Tofu

Total Time: 1 hour 30 mins / **Prep. Time:** 1 hour 10 mins /**Cooking Time:** 20 mins /**Difficulty:** Easy /**Serving Size:** 4 servings

Ingredients:

- 14 oz. water-packed tofu, drained
- 2/3 cup lime juice
- 6 tbsp. toasted sesame oil
- 2/3 cup soy sauce, low sodium

Instructions:

To prepare the tofu, pat it dry and cut it into 1/2 inch cubes. In a medium bowl or big sealable plastic bag, combine the lime juice, soy sauce, and oil. Toss in the tofu lightly to mix. Marinate for 1 hour in the refrigerator, carefully stirring once or twice. Preheat the oven to 450°F. Using a slotted spoon, remove the tofu from the marinade. Place the pieces on two big baking sheets, ensuring they don't touch. Roast carefully turning halfway through, for about 20 minutes, or until golden brown.

Nutritional Values: Calories: 163 kcal /Carbohydrates: 2 g /Protein: 19 g /Fat: 11 g/Sodium: 111 mg

Tomato Cheese Toast

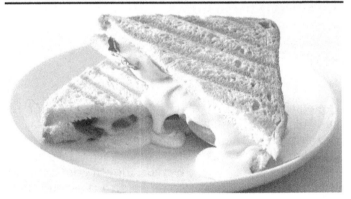

Total Time: 7 mins / **Prep. Time:** 5 mins /**Cooking Time:** 2 mins /**Difficulty:** Easy

Serving Size: 1 serving

Ingredients:

- 1 diagonal slice baguette, whole-wheat
- 1½ tbsp. Cheddar cheese, shredded
- pinch of black pepper
- 2 small slices tomato

Instructions:

Add cheese, tomato, and pepper to toasted bread. If preferred, melt the cheese in a toaster oven (or broil).

Nutritional Values: Calories: 80 kcal /Carbohydrates: 8 g /Protein: 4 g /Fat: 4 g/Sodium: 138 mg

Caprese Skewers

Total Time: 10 mins / **Prep. Time:** 10 mins /**Cooking Time:** N/A /**Difficulty:** Easy

Serving Size: 16 servings

Ingredients:

- 16 fresh mozzarella balls
- 16 cherry tomatoes
- Extra-virgin olive oil, to drizzle
- 16 fresh basil leaves
- salt to taste
- freshly ground pepper, to taste

Instructions:

On tiny skewers, thread tomatoes, basil and mozzarella. Sprinkle with pepper and salt after drizzling with oil.

Nutritional Values: Calories: 46 kcal /Carbohydrates: 1 g /Protein: 3 g /Fat: 2 g/Sodium: 216 mg

Avocado and Salsa Cracker

Total Time: 5 mins / **Prep. Time:** 5 mins /**Cooking Time:** N/A /**Difficulty:** Easy

Serving Size: 1 serving

Ingredients:

- ⅛ avocado
- 1 tbsp. low-sodium salsa
- 1 tbsp. cilantro, for garnish
- 1 large whole-grain crispbread

Instructions:

In a small bowl, mash the avocado, then spread it on the crispbread. Serve with salsa on the top. Garnish with cilantro and enjoy.

Nutritional Values: Calories: 76 kcal /Carbohydrates: 2 g /Protein: 1 g /Fat: 4 g/Sodium: 138 mg

Deviled Eggs

Total Time: 20 mins / **Prep. Time:** 10 mins /**Cooking Time:** 12 mins/**Difficulty:** Easy /**Serving Size:** 24 servings

Ingredients:

- 12 eggs
- 2 tbsp. chopped chives
- ½ cup mayonnaise
- 2 tsp. Dijon mustard
- black pepper to taste
- salt to taste
- paprika for garnish

Instructions:

Boil the eggs in boiling water for 12 minutes. After boiling them place them in ice cold water and peel them. Slice the eggs and cut them in half lengthwise. Half of the yolks should be discarded, and the remaining should be placed in a small bowl. With a fork, thoroughly mash the yolks. Combine chives, mayonnaise, and mustard in a mixing bowl. Add salt and pepper to taste. Fill the hollows in the egg whites with the prepared mixture and sprinkle with paprika. Arrange on a serving dish and serve.

Nutritional Values: Calories: 30 kcal /Carbohydrates: 1 g /Protein: 3 g /Fat: 2 g/Sodium: 76 mg

Lemon Tuna and Yogurt Cracker

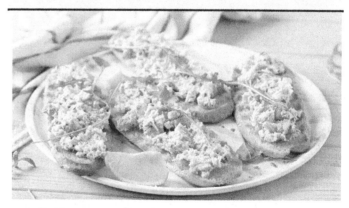

Total Time: 10 mins / **Prep. Time:** 10 mins /**Cooking Time:** N/A /**Difficulty:** Easy

Serving Size: 2 servings

Ingredients:

- 2 tbsp. chunk-light tuna
- ¼ tsp. lemon zest
- 2 large crispbread, whole-grain
- 2 tbsp. plain Greek yogurt, low-fat
- 1 tsp. dill, for garnish

Instructions:

In a small bowl, combine the yogurt, tuna, and lemon zest. Spread the mixture on top of the crispbread.

Garnish with dill and enjoy.

Nutritional Values: Calories: 77 kcal /Carbohydrates: 8 g /Protein: 10 g /Fat: 0.4 g/Sodium: 45 mg

Spiced Crackers

Total Time: 25 mins / **Prep. Time:** 15 mins /**Cooking Time:** 10 mins /**Difficulty:** Easy /**Serving Size:** 8 servings

Ingredients:

- 3 cups whole-grain crackers
- 3 tbsp. olive oil
- 1½ tsp. dried oregano
- 1½ tsp. ground paprika
- pinch of salt

Instructions:

Preheat the oven to 300°F. In a large mixing bowl, combine the paprika, oil, oregano, and salt. Toss in the crackers to coat. Place on a lined baking sheet. Bake 10 minutes in the preheated oven. Allow it cool for 10 minutes on the pan.

Nutritional Values: Calories: 114 kcal /Carbohydrates: 10 g /Protein: 2 g /Fat: 7 g/Sodium: 140 mg

Roasted Flavored

Chickpeas

Total Time: 35 mins / **Prep. Time:** 5 mins /**Cooking Time:** 30 mins /**Difficulty:** Easy /**Serving Size:** 6 servings

Ingredients:

- 2 cups tin can chickpeas
- ½ tsp. ground cumin
- 2 tsp. rapeseed oil

Instructions:

Rinse the chickpeas before patting them dry with paper towels. Preheat the oven to 400°F. Grease the baking tray using 1 tsp. of rapeseed oil and put the tray in pre-heated oven for 3 minutes. Arrange the chickpeas in heated tray and cook for 15 minutes, stirring a number of times to ensure equal cooking of the chickpeas on the hot baking surface. Remove the chickpeas from the oven and pour them in a dish with the remaining oil. Mix thoroughly. Chilli powder and Cumin and cumin should be added now. Re-mix and return to the baking sheet. Cook for another 10-15

minutes, or until golden brown and crisp. Serve immediately or allow cooling before eating.

Nutritional Values: Calories: 62 kcal /Carbohydrates: 0 g /Protein: 3 g /Fat: 2 g/Sodium: 200 mg

Hummus

Total Time: 5 mins / **Prep. Time:** 5 mins /**Cooking Time:** N/A /**Difficulty:** Easy

Serving Size: 3 servings

Ingredients:

- 1 cup tinned chickpeas
- 1 clove garlic
- 2 tsp. lemon juice
- ¼ cup tahini
- ½ cup water
- Salt to taste
- ½ tsp. black pepper

Instructions:

In a blender, blend the chickpeas, tahini, lemon juice, garlic, pepper and salt. To form a firm paste, add a little water. The amount of water you'll need may vary, so start with a little amount and work your way up. You may also add some olive oil for a richer flavour, but remember that more oil means more calories.

Nutritional Values: Calories: 188 kcal /Carbohydrates: 10 g /Protein: 8 g /Fat: 12 g/Sodium: 100 mg

Sweet Potato Crisps

Total Time: 20 mins / **Prep. Time:** 5 mins /**Cooking Time:** 15 mins /**Difficulty:** Easy /**Serving Size:** 8 servings

Ingredients:

- 500g sweet potatoes
- 2 tbsp. vegetable oil

Instructions:

Use a sharp knife or potato slicer to peel a sweet potato and cut it into extremely thin slices. Toss the sweet potato pieces with vegetable oil in a mixing dish. Cover the base of a baking tray with aluminium foil and arrange the sweet potato slices on top. Roast for 10 to 15 minutes, until crispy, before serving.

Nutritional Values: Calories: 73 kcal /Carbohydrates: 10 g /Protein: 1 g /Fat: 3 g/Sodium:

0 mg

Bruschetta

Total Time: 5 mins / **Prep. Time:** 2 mins
/**Cooking Time:** 3 mins /**Difficulty:** Easy

Serving Size: 4 servings

Ingredients:

- 4 slices crusty wholegrain bread
- 2 tsp. olive oil
- ½ clove garlic
- 2 medium tomatoes

Instructions:

Lightly brush each piece of bread with 1/2 tsp. olive oil. Place the pieces under the grill, making sure they don't overcook. Place the cut face of the garlic against the bread and lightly massage it in. Chop the tomatoes and mi with remaining olive oil and arrange them on the cooked bread slices. Enjoy your meal.

Nutritional Values: Calories: 101 kcal /Carbohydrates: 14 g /Protein: 4 g /Fat: 2 g/Sodium: 200 mg

Quick Pizza

Total Time: 50 mins / **Prep. Time:** 15 mins
/**Cooking Time:** 35 mins /**Difficulty:** Medium
/**Serving Size:** 4 servings

Ingredients:

- ½ cup low-fat margarine
- 1 cup self-raising white flour
- 1 medium onion, sliced
- 4 button mushrooms, sliced
- ¼ cup low-fat cheddar cheese, grated
- 1 tbsp. semi-skimmed milk
- 14oz. chopped tomatoes, canned

Instructions:

In a frying pan, add the tomatoes. Add the onion and mushrooms to the tomatoes and cook for 5 minutes on low heat. In a mixing bowl, sieve the flour. Margarine should be rubbed in the flour. Mix in the milk until you have a firm ball. Roll into a huge ball with a thickness of half inch. Place on a prepared baking sheet. Spread the prepared tomato mixture on the bottom, and then top with cheese. Preheat the oven to 350°F and bake for 30 minutes, or until the crust is golden brown.

Nutritional Values: Calories: 398 kcal /Carbohydrates: 5 g /Protein: 11 g /Fat: 20 g/Sodium: 300 mg

Chapter 16: Soups

Soup is a quick and easy meal to prepare ahead of time, and it's a fantastic way to include some healthy and fiber-rich vegetables into your diet. The more vegetables you can consume, the healthier for persons with diabetes. Vegetables are high in vitamins, antioxidants, minerals, and even fiber, all of which your body requires. Most vegetables are also low calorie and carbohydrates, making them ideal for diabetics.

Soups made with pulses and vegetables may be a full and healthy supper. Soups with lentils, for example, may keep you satiated for longer than consuming the same items individually.

Soup is an excellent choice if you have diabetes and want to avoid eating in between meals. Here in this chapter are some healthy soup recipes for persons with type-2 diabetes.

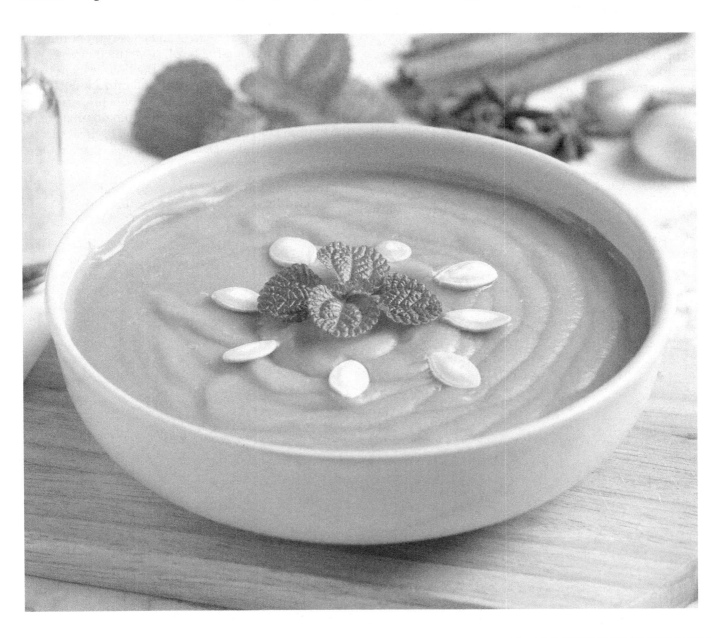

Cauliflower Almond Soup

Total Time: 35 mins / **Prep. Time:** 10 mins /**Cooking Time:** 25 mins /**Difficulty:** Medium/**Serving Size:** 4 servings

Ingredients:

- 2 tbsp. almond oil
- 1 leek, light green and white parts, sliced
- 2 stalks celery, chopped
- 4 cups cauliflower florets
- 1 quart chicken broth, low-sodium
- ¾ tsp. kosher salt
- ¼ tsp. ground nutmeg
- ¼ tsp. black pepper
- ¾ cup almond-cashew cream
- ½ cup sliced almonds, toasted
- ¼ cup chopped parsley

Instructions:

In a large soup pot, heat the almond oil over medium heat. Add celery and cook, stirring occasionally, until the celery begins to soften. Now add the leak and cook until both vegetables are tender. Set aside a few cauliflower florets for garnish after steaming them and add the remaining cauliflower to the vegetable mixture. Add stock, pepper, salt, nutmeg to the vegetables mixture and boil it. Cook the soup for about 10 minutes, or until the cauliflower is tender. In a food processor or blender, puree the soup. Add the almond-cashew cream and mix well. Garnish each soup serving with1 tbsp. parsley, 2 tbsp. almonds, and a few reserved cauliflower florets and serve warm.

Nutritional Values: Calories: 195 kcal /Carbohydrates: 14 g /Protein: 7 g /Fat: 14 g/Sodium: 274 mg

Butternut Squash and Millet Soup

Total Time: 45 mins / **Prep. Time:** 20 mins /**Cooking Time:** 25 mins /**Difficulty:** Medium/**Serving Size:** 6 servings

Ingredients:

- 1 red bell pepper
- 2 ¼ cups butternut squash, diced
- 1 tsp. canola oil
- 1 medium red onion, chopped
- ½ tsp. smoked paprika
- 1 tsp. curry powder
- 1/ tsp. black pepper
- 2 cups chicken broth, low-sodium
- ½ tsp. salt
- 4 oz. chicken breasts, cooked and chopped
- 1 cup cooked millet

Instructions:

Place bell pepper on shelf in broiler pan 3–5 inches away from heating element or use long-handled metal fork to hold over open gas flame. Turn the bell pepper periodically until both sides are blistered and browned. Place the charred bell pepper in the food storage bag and let aside for 15 to 20 minutes to release the skin. With a paring knife, remove any loose skin. Remove the top and scrape out the seeds before discarding. In a large saucepan, heat the oil over high heat. Cook and stir for 5 minutes with the bell pepper, butternut squash, and onion. Combine the curry powder, salt, paprika, and black pepper in a mixing bowl. Add the broth and bring to a boil. Cook for 7 to 10 minutes, or until vegetables are cooked, covered. Purée the soup in batches in a food processor or blender or puree it in a saucepan with a hand-held immersion blender. Return the soup to the pan. Cook, stirring constantly, until the chicken and millet are well cooked.

Nutritional Values: Calories: 168 kcal /Carbohydrates: 19 g /Protein: 16 g /Fat: 3 g/Sodium: 199 mg

Avocado Summer Soup

Total Time: 25 mins / **Prep. Time:** 20 mins /**Cooking Time:** 5 mins /**Difficulty:** Easy /**Serving Size:** 8 servings

Ingredients:

- 1 small onion, finely chopped
- 1 tbsp. canola oil
- 1 garlic clove, minced
- ¼ cup lime juice
- 2 ripe avocados
- 2 tbsp. sherry
- ½ tsp. hot pepper sauce
- 14 oz. chicken stock, low-sodium
- 2 tbsp. fresh cilantro, chopped
- Dash kosher salt
- 2 cups milk, low-fat

Instructions:

In a skillet sauté the garlic and onions till tender and aromatic. The avocado should be peeled and chopped. Purée the garlic and onion blend, lime juice, and sherry in a food processor or blender. Transfer this soup into the mixing bowl. Combine the hot sauce and chicken broth in the prepared soup and blend until smooth. Add the milk and chopped cilantro in the soup. Before serving, season with salt and refrigerate for 2 to 3 hours. More chopped cilantro can be used as a garnish.

Nutritional Values: Calories: 125 kcal /Carbohydrates: 9 g /Protein: 4 g /Fat: 9 g/Sodium: 50 mg

Broccoli Soup

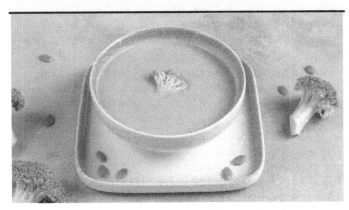

Total Time: 30 mins / **Prep. Time:** 10 mins /**Cooking Time:** 20 mins /**Difficulty:** Easy /**Serving Size:** 6 servings

Ingredients:

- 4 cups vegetable or chicken broth
- 1 onion, quartered
- 2½ lb. broccoli florets
- 1 cup milk, low-fat
- ¼ cup blue cheese, crumbled
- ¼ tsp. salt

Instructions:

In a large saucepan, combine the broccoli, broth, and onion; bring to a boil above high heat. After a boil r educe to a low heat setting, cover, and cook for 20 minutes, or until vegetables are soft. In a blender, puree the soup and return it to the pot. Add milk and salt to the soup. If necessary, add more broth or water. Pour the soup into serving dishes and top with cheese.

Nutritional Values: Calories: 91 kcal /Carbohydrates: 12 g /Protein: 7 g /Fat: 2 g/Sodium: 175 mg

Pumpkin and Green Chile Soup

Total Time: 30 mins / **Prep. Time:** 20 mins /**Cooking Time:** 10 mins /**Difficulty:** Medium/**Serving Size:** 4 servings

Ingredients:

- 4 oz. mild green chile, diced
- ¼ cup fresh cilantro leaves
- ¼ cup light sour cream
- 14 oz. vegetable or chicken broth, low sodium
- 15 oz. solid-pack pumpkin
- 1 tsp. ground cumin
- ½ cup water
- ¼ tsp. garlic powder
- ½ tsp. chili powder
- 1/8 tsp. ground red pepper

Instructions:

In a food processor or blender, puree the chiles with 1/4 cup sour cream, and cilantro until smooth. In a medium saucepan, combine the broth, pumpkin, water, cumin, chilli powder, red pepper and garlic powder; whisk in 1/4 cup green chile mixture. Bring to a boil, and then lower to a low heat setting. Cook for 5 minutes, uncovered, stirring periodically. Fill four serving bowls halfway with soup; top each with tiny dollops of leftover green chile mixture and more sour cream, if preferred. To swirl, run the tip of a spoon through the dollops.

Nutritional Values: Calories: 72 kcal /Carbohydrates: 12 g /Protein: 4 g /Fat: 1 g/Sodium: 276 mg

Vegetable lentil soup

Total Time: 1 hour 10 mins / **Prep. Time:** 15 mins /**Cooking Time:** 55 mins /**Difficulty:** Medium/**Serving Size:** 4 servings

Ingredients:

- Nonstick cooking spray
- ½ cup chopped onion
- 2 medium carrots, thinly sliced
- 4 cups water
- 2 tsp. chicken bouillon
- ¾ cup dried lentils
- 4 cups water
- 2 tsp. chicken bouillon
- ¾ cup dried lentils

- 1/8 tsp. ground red pepper
- ½ tsp. ground cumin
- 1 medium tomato, diced
- 2 tsp. olive oil
- ½ cup roasted red bell peppers, chopped
- ¼ tsp. salt
- 2 tbsp. fresh cilantro, chopped

Instructions:

Spray a large pot with cooking spray and heat over medium-high heat. Cook and stir carrots and onion for 4 minutes or until onion are transparent. Water, bouillon, lentils, red pepper and cumin are added to the pot at this stage. Over high heat, bring to a boil and then r Reduce the heat to low, cover, and cook for 45 minutes, or until the lentils are very soft. Remove from the heat and add the peppers, tomato, oil, and salt to taste. Before serving, cover and set aside for 5 minutes. Serve with cilantro as a garnish.

Nutritional Values: Calories: 182 kcal /Carbohydrates: 29 g /Protein: 11 g /Fat: 3 g/Sodium: 466 mg

White Bean Soup

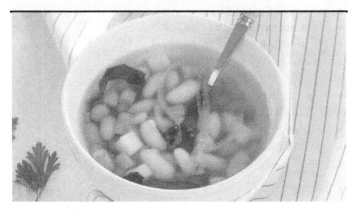

Total Time: 45 mins / **Prep. Time:** 15 mins /**Cooking Time:** 25-30 mins /**Difficulty:** Medium /**Serving Size:** 6 servings

Ingredients:

- 1 cup dried white beans, soaked overnight
- 1 large onion, chopped
- 1 tbsp. canola oil
- freshly ground pepper
- 3 stalks celery, chopped
- ½ tsp. dried sage
- 4 cups vegetable stock or water
- basil pesto
- 1 cup diced tomatoes
- salt to taste

- 1–2 cups fresh spinach, chopped
- freshly grated Parmesan cheese

Instructions:

Beans should be drained. In a pressure cooker, heat the canola oil and add the drained beans, celery, onion, and some fresh pepper. Cook for approximately 5 minutes, until the veggies and beans are aromatic. Add the stock or water, as well as the sage. Secure the cover and raise the pressure to high. Cooking time is 20 minutes. Allow for gradual pressure release after turning off the heat. Remove the cover and toss in the tomatoes and spinach. Cook until the spinach is tender. Season the soup with salt and freshly ground pepper to taste. Serve with a dollop of basil pesto or freshly grated Parmesan cheese.

Nutritional Values: Calories: 162 kcal /Carbohydrates: 28 g /Protein: 9 g /Fat: 3 g/Sodium: 230 mg

Winter Squash Soup

Total Time: 30 mins / **Prep. Time:** 10 mins /**Cooking Time:** 20 mins /**Difficulty:** Medium/**Serving Size:** 4 servings

Ingredients:

- 1½ cups winter squash, cooked and mashed
- dash nutmeg
- 2 tbsp. light margarine
- 1 small onion, finely chopped
- 2 cups chicken broth, fat-free
- 1 tbsp. all-purpose flour
- 1 tsp. dill
- ¼ cup skim milk
- ½ tsp. thyme leaves

Instructions:

In a medium pot, melt margarine and sauté onion. When the onions have softened, add the flour. Slowly pour in a few ounces of chicken broth at a time, stirring frequently. Bring the soup to a moderate boil. Reduce the heat to low and slowly mix in the mashed squash and milk. Season the soup with salt and pepper. Cook for 10 minutes, stirring occasionally. Serve warm and enjoy.

Nutritional Values: Calories: 113 kcal /Carbohydrates: 15 g /Protein: 2 g /Fat: 5 g/Sodium: 508 mg

Keto Vegetable Soup

Total Time: 30 mins / **Prep. Time:** 10 mins /**Cooking Time:** 20 mins /**Difficulty:** Medium/**Serving Size:** 4 servings

Ingredients:

- 2 tbsp. olive oil
- 1 clove garlic, minced
- ½ small onion, diced
- 1 tbsp. tomato paste
- 2 stalks celery, diced
- 1 cup green beans, chopped
- 3 cups vegetable stock
- 2 tsp. Italian seasoning
- 1 cup broccoli, chopped
- 2 cups baby spinach

Instructions:

Heat the olive oil in a big saucepan over medium heat. When the oil is heated, add the garlic, onion, and celery, and sauté, turning regularly, for approximately 2-3 minutes, or until the onion begins to soften. Cook for a further 1-2 minutes after adding the Italian seasoning and tomato paste. Combine the broccoli, green beans, and vegetable stock in a large mixing bowl. Bring to a gentle boil, then reduce to a low heat and cook for 10-15 minutes, or until the beans are tender. Add the spinach and mix well. Remove from the heat and serve immediately.

Nutritional Values: Calories: 109 kcal /Carbohydrates: 7 g /Protein: 2 g /Fat: 8 g/Sodium: 58 mg

Vegan Mushroom Soup

Total Time: 40 mins / **Prep. Time:** 10 mins /**Cooking Time:** 30 mins /**Difficulty:** Medium /**Serving Size:** 4 servings

Ingredients:

- 1 tsp. olive oil
- 1 clove fresh garlic
- 1 large onion, diced
- 8 sprigs fresh thyme
- 16 oz. mushrooms
- 1 tbsp. coconut Aminos
- 14 oz. canned coconut milk
- 2 cups vegetable broth, low-sodium
- Salt and pepper to taste

Instructions:

Chop the garlic, onions, and mushrooms into small pieces. In a large saucepan over medium heat, combine the oil, garlic, onion, and mushrooms. Cook for a further 8–10 minutes, or until the mushrooms begin to release their juices. Stir in the other ingredients until well combined. Bring the soup to a boiling point, then lower to a low heat and continue to cook for 15 minutes. Fill a food processor or blender halfway with soup. Blend until completely smooth, and then return to the soup pot. This adds additional creaminess to the soup. To serve, garnish with coconut milk and fresh thyme sprigs.

Nutritional Values: Calories: 221 kcal /Carbohydrates: 13 g /Protein: 3 g /Fat: 16 g/Sodium: 152 mg

Coconut Chicken Soup

Total Time: 50 mins / **Prep. Time:** 20 mins /**Cooking Time:** 30 mins /**Difficulty:** Hard/**Serving Size:** 6 servings

Ingredients:

- 1 lb. chicken breast, sliced
- 1 tbsp. coconut oil
- Salt and pepper, to taste
- 2 garlic cloves, minced
- 1 small onion, thinly sliced
- 1 medium zucchini, diced
- 1 inch piece ginger, minced
- 1 red bell pepper, thinly sliced
- 1 cup pumpkin, cubed
- 14 oz. lite coconut milk
- 1 small chili pepper, thinly sliced
- Juice of 1 lime
- 2 cups chicken broth
- Handful cilantro leaves

Instructions:

Marinate the sliced chicken breast with salt and pepper to taste. Heat the coconut oil in a large soup pot over high heat before adding the chicken breast. Add marinated chicken and stir-fry for 4-5 minutes over high heat, or until the surface of the chicken is no longer pink. Combine the chopped onion, minced ginger and garlic in the pot and stir-fry for a further 2-3 minutes. Stir in the chopped zucchini and cubed pumpkin. Add the sliced chilli pepper, bell pepper, chicken broth, coconut milk, and lime juice and give everything a thorough stir once more. Bring to a boil, then reduce to a low heat, cover, and cook for 20 minutes, just until the pumpkin is completely cooked. Remove from the heat and, if needed, season with more salt and pepper. Before serving garnish the soup with cilantro leaves.

Nutritional Values: Calories: 231 kcal /Carbohydrates: 12 g /Protein: 17 g /Fat: 13 g/Sodium: 45 mg

Squash and Cauliflower Soup

Total Time: 30 mins / **Prep. Time:** 10 mins /**Cooking Time:** 20 mins /**Difficulty:** Medium /**Serving Size:** 4 servings

Ingredients:

- 2 tablespoon olive oil
- 3 cloves garlic, minced
- ½ yellow onion, diced
- 2 ½ cups cauliflower florets
- 1 tbsp. fresh ginger, minced
- ½ tsp. ground cardamom
- 2 ½ cups squash, cubed
- 2 bay leaves
- ¼ tsp. cayenne
- 4 cups chicken broth
- ½ tsp. salt
- ½ cup vanilla almond milk, unsweetened
- ¼ tsp. pepper

Instructions:

In a large saucepan warm the olive oil over medium heat. Add the garlic, onion, and ginger in the pan and sauté for 3 minutes, or until onions start to turn translucent and aromatic. Mix the cauliflower, cardamom, squash, bay leaves and cayenne in the pot and stir everything together, and then pour in the broth. Bring the mixture to a boil, and then reduce to a low heat. Cook for about 10 minutes, or until a fork can easily pierce the squash. Puree the ingredients in a high-powered blender or in your cooking pot using an immersion blender. Return the soup to the pot over low heat after it has been smoothly blended. Season the soup with salt and pepper after adding the almond milk. Serve warm and enjoy.

Nutritional Values: Calories: 125 kcal /Carbohydrates: 12 g /Protein: 3 g /Fat: 8 g/Sodium: 1185 mg

Zucchini Soup

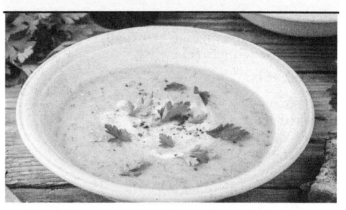

Total Time: 50 mins / **Prep. Time:** 10 mins /**Cooking Time:** 40 mins /**Difficulty:** Medium/**Serving Size:** 4 servings

Ingredients:

- 4 medium sized zucchinis
- 2-3 cloves garlic
- 1 medium onion
- 2 tbsp. tapioca flour
- 2 cups chicken stock
- ¼ tsp. salt
- ½ tsp. black pepper
- 8 slices turkey bacon, low-fat
- 4 tbsp. fresh parsley
- 4 hardboiled eggs
- cooking spray

Instructions:

Cut the onion and zucchini into large pieces and cut the garlic cloves in half. Cook the vegetables in a big saucepan with a little cooking spray for 5-10 minutes over medium heat, stirring every few of minutes. Add chicken stock in the vegetables and allow 20 minutes for the chicken stock to boil with the vegetables. Add all of the ingredients in a blender or blend everything in the saucepan using a stick blender. Whisk in the tapioca flour with the soup. When the flour is thoroughly incorporated, season with salt & pepper and continue to cook for another 10 minutes. Meanwhile Cook the bacon till it is crisp. Serve the soup with a garnish of chopped boiled eggs, parsley and bacon on top.

Nutritional Values: Calories: 290 kcal /Carbohydrates: 32 g /Protein: 16 g /Fat: 11 g/Sodium: 200 mg

Golden Soup

Total Time: 45 mins / **Prep. Time:** 15 mins /**Cooking Time:** 30 mins /**Difficulty:** Medium/**Serving Size:** 6 servings

Ingredients:

- 1 red onion
- 1 red pepper
- 1 white onion
- 2 large courgettes
- 2 yellow peppers
- ¼ tsp. dry mixed herbs
- 2 tomatoes
- Cooking spray
- 1 low-salt stock cube
- 1 tsp. nutritional yeast
- 3 cups boiling water

Instructions:

Preheat oven to 425°F. To speed up the roasting process, chop all the vegetables into bits, sprinkle with nutritional yeast and dry mixed herbs, and spritz with oil of choice.   Place in the centre of the oven for 25–30 minutes, or until the vegetables are browned and bronzed around the edges. Separately, dissolve the stock in warm water and set aside until ready to use in the Blitzer. Stir and blitz until smooth, then pour into a pan to reheat. Serve once you've double-checked the seasoning.

Nutritional Values: Calories: 63 kcal /Carbohydrates: 9 g /Protein: 2 g /Fat: 1 g/Sodium: 90 mg

Black Bean and Chorizo Soup

Total Time: 50 mins / **Prep. Time:** 10 mins /**Cooking Time:** 35 mins /**Difficulty:** Easy /**Serving Size:** 10 servings

Ingredients:

- 1 tbsp. canola oil
- 1 clove garlic, minced
- ½ onion, cubed
- 1 ancho chile
- 1 tomato, deseeded and chopped
- 6 tbsp. chorizo,crumbled
- 1 can black beans
- 1 pasilla pepper
- 1 tbsp. oregano,

- 1 tbsp. dried cilantro
- 4 cup chicken broth
- 1 lime, halved
- Salt to taste
- 2 tbsp. tequila

Instructions:

Heat canola oil in a deep skillet or pot over high heat, and then add onion. Cook till brown, and then add the garlic. Reduce to a medium heat setting. Stir in peppers and tomatoes. Cook for 15 minutes, continually stirring to avoid scorching. Mix in the black beans, cilantro, oregano, limes, and broth. After 5 minutes of cooking add salt, mezcal or tequila, and discard lime halves and herbs. Cook for another ten minutes. Blend the soup and garnish with chorizo and buttermilk.

Nutritional Values: Calories: 180 kcal /Carbohydrates: 18 g /Protein: 10 g /Fat: 7 g/Sodium: 310 mg

Pumpkin Soup

Total Time: 1 our 20 mins / **Prep. Time:** 10 mins /**Cooking Time:** 1 hour 10 mins /**Difficulty:** Medium /**Serving Size:** 8 servings

Ingredients:

- 4 cups pumpkin puree
- 4 cups vegetable broth, divided
- 1 clove garlic
- 1 cup onion, finely chopped
- Salt and black pepper to taste
- 1 tsp. fresh thyme, chopped
- Nutmeg, for garnish
- 2 tbsp. light whipping cream
- 1 tsp. fresh parsley, chopped

Instructions:

Add pumpkin puree, 3 cups broth, garlic, onion, thyme, salt, and pepper in a large saucepan over medium-high heat. Bring the soup to a boil. Reduce to a low heat and cook for 30 minutes, uncovered. In small batches, puree the contents in a food processor or blender until smooth. Return the pot to its original state. Reduce to a low heat and continue to cook, uncovered, for another 30 minutes. As needed, add the remaining broth. Fill bowls with the mixture. Serve with parsley and nutmeg sprinkling on top.

Nutritional Values: Calories: 71 kcal /Carbohydrates: 16 g /Protein: 3 g /Fat: 1 g/Sodium: 284 mg

Spinach and Onion Soup

Total Time: 30 mins / **Prep. Time:** 10 mins /**Cooking Time:** 20 mins /**Difficulty:** Easy /**Serving Size:** 4 servings

Ingredients:

- 6 cups spinach leaves
- 2 medium onions, thinly sliced
- 1 tbsp. vegetable oil
- 1 bay leaf
- 4 cups vegetable stock
- 2/3 cup white wine
- Salt and pepper, to taste

Instructions:

In a skillet, heat the oil and cook the onions for around 5-8 minutes over low heat, until tender. Bring the stock to a boil, and then remove from the heat. Season the soup with the bay leaf and spices. Cook for 10 minutes with the lid on. Pour the wine in and toss in the spinach. Cook for another minute or two, till the spinach has wilted little. Remove the bay leaf before serving.

Nutritional Values: Calories: 141 kcal /Carbohydrates: 14 g /Protein: 6 g /Fat: 6 g/Sodium: 1011 mg

Tomato Soup

Total Time: 55 mins / **Prep. Time:** 10 mins /**Cooking Time:** 45 mins /**Difficulty:** Medium/**Serving Size:** 4 servings

Ingredients:

- 1 tbsp. butter
- 2 large garlic cloves, chopped
- 1 onion, finely chopped
- 1 tbsp. sugar
- 28 oz. diced tomatoes
- 1/8 tsp. ground mace
- 1 tsp. dried thyme
- ½ cup half-and-half cream, fat-free
- Pinch of cayenne pepper
- 3 tbsp. snipped dill, for garnish
- Salt and black pepper, to taste

Instructions:

In a small Dutch oven, melt the butter over medium-high heat. Cook the onions for 4 minutes until they are transparent. Add the garlic and sauté for next 5 to 6 minutes. Toss in the tomatoes and their juices, as well as the thyme, sugar, mace, and cayenne pepper.

Bring to a boil, then reduce to a low heat and cook for 15 minutes, or until the onion and tomatoes are tender. Allow the soup to rest, uncovered, for 20 minutes. Transfer the mixture to a blender and purée it to your preferred consistency, either pulpy or entirely smooth. Blend cream with the soup and season the soup with salt and pepper to taste. Sprinkle dill over each bowl before serving.

Nutritional Values: Calories: 105 kcal /Carbohydrates: 18 g /Protein: 3 g /Fat: 3 g/Sodium: 586 mg

Chickpea Soup

Total Time: 30 mins / **Prep. Time:** 5 mins /**Cooking Time:** 25 mins /**Difficulty:** Easy /**Serving Size:** 6 servings

Ingredients:

- 1 tsp. olive oil
- 1 garlic clove, minced
- 1 small onion, chopped
- 1 carrot, sliced
- 1 celery stalk, sliced
- 1 cup plum tomatoes with liquid
- ½ red bell pepper, diced
- 1 cup canned chickpeas, rinsed, drained
- ½ tsp. dried leaf basil
- 4 cups Chicken Broth
- Black pepper to taste

Instructions:

Heat the oil in a nonstick skillet and sauté the garlic, onion, and celery for 5 minutes. Mix together the remaining ingredients. Bring to a boil, and then lower to a low heat and cook, covered, for 20 minutes.

Nutritional Values: Calories: 74 kcal /Carbohydrates: 13 g /Protein: 5 g /Fat: 1 g/Sodium: 96 mg

Mushroom Soup

Total Time: 35 mins / **Prep. Time:** 15 mins /**Cooking Time:** 20 mins /**Difficulty:** Medium/**Serving Size:** 6 servings

Ingredients:

- ½ cup chopped onion
- 1 lb. mushrooms, thinly sliced
- 3 strips bacon, diced
- 6 cups chicken broth

- 1/3 cup all-purpose flour
- 1 small packet chicken bouillon granules
- 1 cup hot water
- 1 tbsp. fresh parsley, chopped
- 2 tbsp. dry sherry
- 1¼ lb. potatoes, peeled and cubed
- ½ cup heavy cream

Instructions:

Cook bacon and onion for 2 to 3 minutes over medium heat in saucepan until onion is brown. Add mushrooms and cook, stirring occasionally, until the liquid has evaporated, about 8 minutes. Now add flour and cook for 1 minute, stirring constantly. In a saucepan, combine broth, water, and bouillon granules. Stir in the sherry and potatoes, and cook for next 15 minutes, or until the potatoes are soft. In a food processor, puree 4 cups of the soup mixture. Return to the pan after pureeing. Add the cream and mix well. Reheat on low to medium heat, stirring periodically. Pour the soup into soup bowls. Serve with parsley as a garnish.

Nutritional Values: Calories: 222 kcal /Carbohydrates: 22 g /Protein: 6 g /Fat: 12 g/Sodium: 435 mg

Chapter 17: Vegetable recipes

Controlling portion sizes and preparing a precise mix of nutrients are the keys to healthy meals for diabetics. People with diabetes may stay healthy while enjoying a variety of meals by eating a broad variety of foods, including a combination of specific vegetables.

Low on the glycemic index scale, high in nitrates, or high in fiber, which lower blood pressure, are the best vegetables for type 2 diabetes. The finest vegetable recipes for patients with type 2 diabetes are discussed in this chapter.

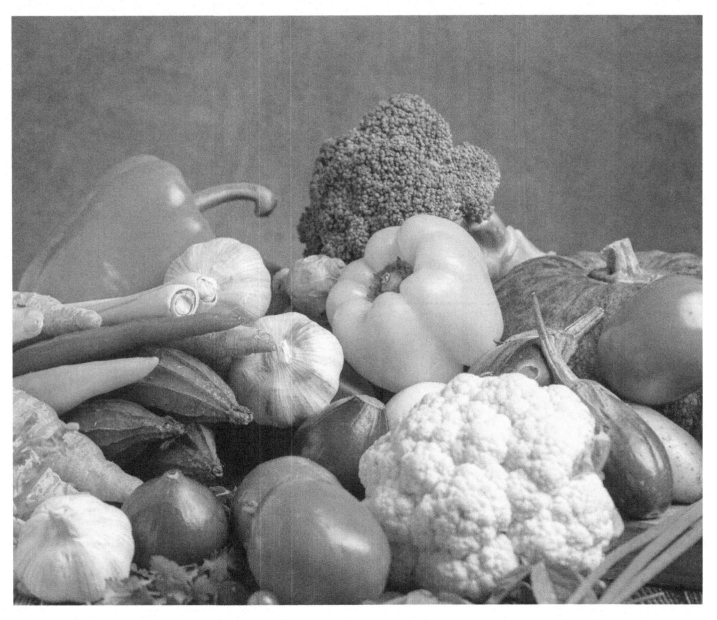

Kale Chips

Total Time: 25 mins / **Prep. Time:** 15 mins /**Cooking Time:** 8-12 mins /**Difficulty:** Easy /**Serving Size:** 4 servings

Ingredients:

- 1 large bunch kale
- ¼ tsp. salt
- 1 tbsp. extra-virgin olive oil

Instructions:

Preheat oven to 400°F, with racks in the upper third and middle. If the kale is moist, thoroughly dry it with a clean kitchen towel before transferring it to a big mixing bowl. Drizzle some oil on the kale and season it with salt. Massage the salt and oil into the kale leaves with your hands until they are uniformly coat. Make a layer of kale on two big rimmed baking pans, ensuring that the leaves don't overlap. Bake until the majority of the leaves are crisp, 8 to 12 minute's total, moving the pans back and forth from front to back and top to bottom halfway through.

Nutritional Values: Calories: 110 kcal /Carbohydrates: 16 g /Protein: 5 g /Fat: 5 g/Sodium: 210 mg

Spinach Rolls

Total Time: 0 mins / **Prep. Time:** 0 mins /**Cooking Time:** 0 mins /**Difficulty:** Easy

Serving Size: 0 servings

Ingredients:

- 16 oz. spinach leaves, frozen
- 2½ oz. onion
- 3 eggs
- 1 oz. low-fat mozzarella cheese
- 2 oz. carrot
- ¾ cup parsley
- 4 oz. fat-free cottage cheese
- 1 tsp. curry powder
- 1 clove garlic
- 1 tsp. salt
- ¼ tsp. chili flakes
- Cooking spray
- 1 tsp. pepper

Instructions:

Preheat the oven to 400°F. Thaw the spinach and drain away any excess liquid. Microwave the spinach for several minutes to allow faster thawing process. In a mixing bowl, combine 2 eggs, spinach, garlic, mozzarella, half the salt, and pepper. Spray a baking sheet with cooking spray and place parchment paper on top. Spread the spinach mixture on the sheet and flatten it to a size of 10*12 inches. Bake the spinach egg mixture for 15 minutes, and then cool on a wire rack. The oven should not be turned off. Chop the onion and parsley finely. Carrots should be grated. Fry the onions in a pan with some cooking spray for approximately a minute. After that, add the parsley and carrots to the pan and cook for about 2 minutes. Add cottage cheese, chilli, curry powder, the remaining half of the salt, and pepper in the pan and mi x for a few seconds. Remove the skillet from the heat, crack an egg into it, and stir everything together. Over the cooled spinach, spread the filling. If you will spread it all the way to the corners, it will flow out so don't spread it near the corners. Roll the spinach sheet and filling carefully, and then bake further for 25 minutes. When the timer goes off, remove the roll and set it aside to cool for 5-10 minutes before slicing and serving.

Nutritional Values: Calories: 310 kcal /Carbohydrates: 19 g /Protein: 27 g /Fat: 10 g/Sodium: 695 mg

Roasted Asparagus with Bacon

Total Time: 20 mins / **Prep. Time:** 5 mins /**Cooking Time:** 15 mins /**Difficulty:** Easy /**Serving Size:** 8 servings

Ingredients:

- 2 lb. fresh asparagus, trimmed
- 12 oz. Bacon, chopped
- 2 tbsp. olive oil

Instructions:

Preheat the oven to 425°F. Combine asparagus, turkey bacon and olive oil in a mixing bowl. Arrange in a single layer. Roast asparagus for 15 minutes, or until crisp tender.

Nutritional Values: Calories: 140 kcal /Carbohydrates: 4 g /Protein: 8 g /Fat: 11 g/Sodium: 370 mg

Brussels sprouts With Tomatoes

Total Time: 25 mins / **Prep. Time:** 5 mins /**Cooking Time:** 20 mins /**Difficulty:** Easy /**Serving Size:** 6 servings

Ingredients:

- 1 lb. Brussels sprouts, trimmed
- 2 tbsp. pure canola oil
- 15 oz. canned tomatoes, drained
- ¼ tsp. salt
- 1/8 tsp. ground black pepper
- ¼ tsp. garlic powder

Instructions:

Preheat the oven to 425°F. Toss drained tomatoes, Brussels sprouts, garlic powder, salt, oil and pepper in a large mixing dish. In a large shallow baking pan, spread the vegetables in a single layer. Bake for 20 minutes, stirring halfway through, or until Brussels sprouts are soft and golden.

Nutritional Values: Calories: 75 kcal /Carbohydrates: 7 g /Protein: 2 g /Fat: 5 g/Sodium: 217 mg

Butternut Squash Crostini

Total Time: 5 mins / **Prep. Time:** 5 mins /**Cooking Time:** N/A /**Difficulty:** Easy

Serving Size: 32 servings

Ingredients:

- 8 slices whole grain bread, toasted
- 4 oz. feta cheese, crumbled
- 2 cups butternut squash, broiled and cubed
- 1 tbsp. fresh thyme leaves
- 2 tbsp. maple syrup
- 32 fresh basil leaves

Instructions:

To make 32 pieces of toast, quarter each slice of bread. In a medium mixing dish, combine the cheese, squash, maple syrup, and thyme. Top each piece of bread with roughly a spoonful of the squash mixture. Garnish with basil leaves.

Nutritional Values: Calories: 30 kcal /Carbohydrates: 5 g /Protein: 1 g /Fat: 1 g/Sodium: 65 mg

Asian Sesame Slaw

Total Time: 10 mins / **Prep. Time:** 10 mins /**Cooking Time:** N/A /**Difficulty:** Easy

Serving Size: 6 servings

Ingredients:

- ½ head of green cabbage, grated
- 6 green onions, sliced diagonally
- ½ head of red cabbage, grated
- 1 tbsp. sesame seeds, toasted
- 1 large carrot, peeled and grated
- ¼ cup canola oil
- 1/3 cup seasoned rice vinegar
- 1 tsp. grated fresh ginger
- 1 garlic clove, minced
- 1 tsp. sesame oil
- 1 tsp. soy sauce, low-sodium

Instructions:

Combine cabbages, carrot, onion, and sesame seeds in a large mixing dish. Shake together canola oil, rice vinegar, ginger, garlic, soy sauce, and sesame oil to make the dressing. Toss the salad with the dressing and chill before serving. Allow about an hour or longer in the refrigerator to allow flavors to meld. Before serving, toss the salad again.

Nutritional Values: Calories: 100 kcal /Carbohydrates: 7 g /Protein: 2 g /Fat: 8 g/Sodium: 170 mg

Garlic Snow Peas with Cilantro

Total Time: 10 mins / **Prep. Time:** 5 mins /**Cooking Time:** 5 mins /**Difficulty:** Easy

Serving Size: 6 servings

Ingredients:

- 3 tsp. canola oil, divided
- 4 medium cloves garlic, minced
- 3 cups snow peas
- ½ cup fresh cilantro, chopped
- ¼ tsp. salt

Instructions:

In a large nonstick pan, heat 1-1/2 tbsp. canola oil in two batches over medium-high heat. Cook for 3 minutes, or until the snow peas are just beginning to brown on the edges, tossing easily with two spoons. Cook for 30 seconds, stirring regularly, after adding half of the garlic. Place on a separate platter and set away. Replace the remaining 1-1/2 tablespoons canola oil, snow peas, and garlic and repeat the process. Return the reserved snow peas to the skillet when done, along with the salt and cilantro, and stir gently but thoroughly. Serve right away to get the most out of the flavors.

Nutritional Values: Calories: 45 kcal /Carbohydrates: 4 g /Protein: 2 g /Fat: 2.5 g/Sodium: 100 mg

Zucchini Parmesan Fritters

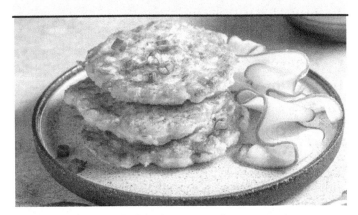

Total Time: 25 mins / **Prep. Time:** 15 mins /**Cooking Time:** 10 mins /**Difficulty:** Medium/**Serving Size:** 6 servings

Ingredients:

- 4 large eggs, separated
- ½ cup grated Parmesan cheese
- 2 medium zucchini, grated
- ¼ cup parsley, chopped
- ½ cup mozzarella cheese, shredded
- ¼ cup coconut-flax flour blend
- ¼ cup fresh basil, chopped
- 1/8 tsp. ground nutmeg
- ½ tsp. baking powder
- cooking spray
- ¼ tsp. salt
- 3 tsp. olive oil

Instructions:

In a large mixing bowl, whisk together the egg whites. Beat on high speed with an electric mixer until firm peaks form and whites cling to the edges of the bowl when tilted. In a separate large mixing bowl, combine the zucchini, egg yolks, mozzarella, Parmesan, basil, parsley, coconut-flax flour blend, nutmeg, baking powder, and salt. Mix vigorously until all of the

zucchini is coated with flour. Carefully f fold in beaten egg whites with a rubber spatula until just blended. There will be egg white streaks. Use cooking spray to coat a big skillet. Heat 1 tsp. oil in a pan over medium-high heat Pour out 4 fritters using a 1/4-cup measuring. Cook until lightly browned on both sides, about 2-3 minutes each side. Place on a platter. Repeat the process twice more, each time using 1 tsp. of oil and four quarter-measures of batter. Serve right away or keep refrigerated, wrapped in aluminium foil, until ready to serve.

Nutritional Values: Calories: 159 kcal /Carbohydrates: 5 g /Protein: 11 g /Fat: 11 g/Sodium: 100 mg

Balsamic Brussels sprouts

Total Time: 20 mins / **Prep. Time:** 10 mins /**Cooking Time:** 10 mins /**Difficulty:** Easy /**Serving Size:** 4 servings

Ingredients:

- 10 oz. Brussels sprouts
- 2 garlic cloves, finely minced
- 2 tbsp. olive oil
- ¼ cup minced red bell pepper
- 2 tbsp. balsamic vinegar
- Salt and black pepper, to taste
- 1 tbsp. parsley, finely chopped

Instructions:

Boil the Brussels sprouts just till soft. Mix together the vinegar, olive oil and garlic. Set aside the dressing. Once the sprouts are done, rinse them carefully and arrange in a shallow serving dish. Dressing should be re-blended and drizzled over sprouts. Sprinkle the parsley and red pepper on top of the sprouts. Season the sprouts with salt and pepper to taste. Serve immediately.

Nutritional Values: Calories: 98 kcal /Carbohydrates: 8 g /Protein: 2 g /Fat: 7 g/Sodium: 195 mg

Broccoli Rabe Sauté

Total Time: 25 mins / **Prep. Time:** 10 mins /**Cooking Time:** 15 mins /**Difficulty:** Easy /**Serving Size:** 8 servings

Ingredients:

- 2 tbsp. canola oil
- 3 large garlic cloves, minced
- 3 bunches broccoli rabe

- 1½ cups roasted red bell pepper, diced
- ½ tsp. salt
- 3 tbsp. slivered almonds, toasted

Instructions:

Over medium-high heat, preheat a very large Dutch oven. Add the rapini, garlic, and salt to the pan with the canola oil. Lower heat to medium-low and put lid after tossing thoroughly. Cook rotating a few times throughout cooking, for 10 minutes just until rapini are soft. Add toasted almonds and roasted pepper, stir and serve.

Nutritional Values: Calories: 110 kcal /Carbohydrates: 11 g /Protein: 7 g /Fat: 5 g/Sodium: 55 mg

Southwestern Roasted Vegetables

Total Time: 50 mins / **Prep. Time:** 10 mins /**Cooking Time:** 40 mins /**Difficulty:** Easy /**Serving Size:** 8 servings

Ingredients:

- 4 cups sweet potatoes, cut 1-inch cubes
- 1 small red onion, small chunks
- 1½ cups zucchini, small chunks
- 3 tbsp. low-sodium taco seasoning mix
- 2 tbsp. olive oil
- 6 oz. portabella mushroom slices, halved
- Salt to taste

Instructions:

Preheat the oven to 425. Line a baking pan with foil or coat it with nonstick cooking spray. Combine zucchini, sweet potatoes, onion, and mushrooms in a large mixing dish. Toss and coat vegetables with olive oil. Spread the coated vegetables on baking sheet and season with taco seasoning and salt. Bake for 40 minutes, tossing the pan every 15 minutes, till soft and roasted.

Nutritional Values: Calories: 110 kcal /Carbohydrates: 17 g /Protein: 2 g /Fat: 4 g/Sodium: 209 mg

Asparagus with Lemon Sauce

Total Time: 22 mins / **Prep. Time:** 15 mins /**Cooking Time:** 7 mins /**Difficulty:** Easy /**Serving Size:** 4 servings

Ingredients:

- 2 tbsp. reduced-fat mayonnaise
- 1 fresh lemon
- 20 medium asparagus spears, trimmed
- 1/8 tsp. ground black pepper
- 1 tbsp. dried parsley
- 1 tsp. salt

Instructions:

In a 4-quart saucepan with a cover, add 1 inch of water. Place asparagus in a steamer basket inside the pot. Bring to a boil, covered, over high heat. Reduce to a medium heat setting. Cook for 7 minutes, or until a sharp knife can easily penetrate through the asparagus. Don't overcook. Grate the lemon zest and squeeze the juice into the mixing bowl. Remove pits and push out excess juice with the back of a spoon. Combine mayonnaise, pepper, parsley, and salt in a mixing bowl. Stir everything together thoroughly. Remove the saucepan from the heat when the asparagus is tender. In a serving bowl, arrange asparagus spears. Serve the asparagus with a drizzle of lemon sauce.

Nutritional Values: Calories: 39 kcal /Carbohydrates: 7 g /Protein: 2 g /Fat: 2 g/Sodium: 107 mg

Parmesan Green Beans

Total Time: 17 mins / **Prep. Time:** 10 mins /**Cooking Time:** 7 mins /**Difficulty:** Easy /**Serving Size:** 4 servings

Ingredients:

- 1 tbsp. olive oil
- 1 small onion, thinly sliced
- 1 tsp garlic, minced
- ¼ tsp. ground black pepper
- 1 cup chicken broth, low-sodium
- 16 oz. frozen green beans
- ¼ cup grated parmesan cheese

Instructions:

In a large saucepan, combine the olive oil and garlic. Cook, stirring occasionally, until the garlic is soft.

Don't overcook the garlic. Add onions and cook for another 5 minutes over medium heat, until the onion is tender. Chicken broth and green beans should be added at this point. Bring to a boil, then reduce to a low heat for 2 minutes, or until the beans are well cooked. Serve with a sprinkling of parmesan cheese and black pepper.

Nutritional Values: Calories: 95 kcal /Carbohydrates: 9 g /Protein: 5 g /Fat: 5 g/Sodium: 117 mg

Jalapeno Broccoli

Total Time: 15 mins / **Prep. Time:** 5 mins /**Cooking Time:** 10 mins /**Difficulty:** Medium/**Serving Size:** 4 servings

Ingredients:

- 1 head broccoli, separated into spears
- 3 tbsp. olive oil
- 1 tbsp. balsamic vinegar
- ¼ cup pine nuts, toasted
- 2 jalapeno peppers, thinly sliced
- Few sprigs parsley, chopped
- Salt to taste

Instructions:

Bring a saucepan of water to a boil and add salt in it. Boil the broccoli spears for 3 to 5 minutes over high heat. Drain broccoli and place it in a dish of ice cold water for few seconds. Drain and arrange the cooked spears on a presentation platter in a creative manner. Drizzle with balsamic vinegar in an even layer. Heat the olive oil in a small frying pan over medium heat for 30 seconds. Stir in the sliced jalapeño peppers and sauté for 2 to 3 minutes, or until softened. Distribute the peppers and all of the oil from the pan equally over the broccoli. Garnish with pine nuts and parsley on top.

Nutritional Values: Calories: 142 kcal /Carbohydrates: 14 g /Protein: 8 g /Fat: 9 g/Sodium: 206 mg

Lemon-Glazed Baby Carrots

Total Time: 15mins / **Prep. Time:** 3 mins /**Cooking Time:** 12 mins /**Difficulty:** Easy /**Serving Size:** 4 servings

Ingredients:

- 1 lb. peeled baby carrots

- 1 tbsp. butter
- 1 tbsp. brown sugar
- ¼ cup vegetable stock
- ½ tsp. grated lemon rind
- 1 tbsp. lemon juice
- ¼ tsp. black pepper
- ¼ tsp. salt
- 1 tbsp. fresh parsley, finely chopped

Instructions:

Cook carrots for 5 to 7 minutes in boiling or until tender-crisp; drain the water and return carrots to pot. Combine the butter, stock, lemon juice, brown sugar, rind, salt, and pepper in the pot of carrots. Cook the carrots for 3 to 5 minutes, stirring often, or until liquid has absorbed and carrots are well coated. Serve with a garnish of parsley.

Nutritional Values: Calories: 91 kcal /Carbohydrates: 15 g /Protein: 2 g /Fat: 3 g/Sodium: 251 mg

Green Beans with Sunflower Seeds

Total Time: 13 mins / **Prep. Time:** 5 mins /**Cooking Time:** 8 mins /**Difficulty:** Easy

Serving Size: 3 servings

Ingredients:

- 1 lb. fresh green beans
- 2 cloves garlic, minced
- ½ cup chopped onion
- 1/8 tsp. black pepper
- ½ tsp. salt
- 2 tbsp. shelled sunflower seeds
- Pinch of red pepper flakes
- ¼ tsp. dried oregano

Instructions:

Snap the beans' ends off. Leave the beans whole if they are very young; if they are large, split them into 2-inch lengths. In a saucepan, combine the beans with 1 cup water, garlic, onion, salt, and pepper. Bring to a boil, then lower to a low heat and cook for approximately 8 minutes, or until the beans are crunchy; drain. Toss the beans with the sunflower seeds and oregano. Toss gently to combine and serve.

Nutritional Values: Calories: 38 kcal /Carbohydrates: 6 g /Protein: 2 g /Fat: 2 g/Sodium: 37 mg

Greek Style Mushrooms

Total Time: 10 mins / **Prep. Time:** 3 mins /**Cooking Time:** 7 mins /**Difficulty:** Easy

Serving Size: 3 servings

Ingredients:

- 1½ lb. mushrooms, stems trimmed flat
- 3 cloves garlic, minced
- ¼ cup red wine vinegar
- 1/3 cup olive oil
- 1 tbsp. whole coriander seeds
- ½ tsp. dried oregano
- ½ tsp. dried thyme
- ½ tsp. freshly ground pepper

Instructions:

In a big sauté pan add garlic and oil and sauté the garlic for 2 minutes. Bring the remaining ingredients to a simmer, except the mushrooms. Add the mushrooms and cook, covered, over low heat for 5 minutes, till soft, stirring occasionally. Fill a glass dish or jar halfway with the mixture. Refrigerate for 1 to 4 days, covered. Before serving, drain and discard the marinade.

Nutritional Values: Calories: 33 kcal /Carbohydrates: 3 g /Protein: 1 g /Fat: 2 g/Sodium: 3 mg

Baby Corn in Jalapeno Vinaigrette

Total Time: 2 hours / **Prep. Time:** 2 hours /**Cooking Time:** N/A /**Difficulty:** Easy

Serving Size: 8 servings

Ingredients:

- 15 oz. whole baby corn cobs
- ¼ cup white wine vinegar
- ¼ cup chopped cilantro
- 1 small jalapeno pepper, minced
- 2 tbsp. olive oil

Instructions:

In a glass dish, combine all of the ingredients and marinate for at least 2 hours or overnight. Before serving drain the corn cobs.

Nutritional Values: Calories: 27 kcal /Carbohydrates: 3 g /Protein: 1 g /Fat: 2 g/Sodium: 5 mg

Cabbage Latkes

Total Time: 16 mins / **Prep. Time:** 10 mins /**Cooking Time:** 6 mins /**Difficulty:** Easy /**Serving Size:** 10 servings

Ingredients:

- 2 cups cabbage, finely grate
- 2 egg whites
- 1 whole egg
- 1 tbsp. canola oil
- 2 tbsp. whole-wheat flour
- salt and pepper to taste
- 1 scallion, chopped
- cooking spray

Instructions:

In a 4-cup dish, place the cabbage. Mix in the scallion and eggs using a wooden spoon. Add flour and season the mixture Season the flour with salt and pepper to taste. Form latkes with damp palms and cook 3 minutes from both sides over medium-high heat.

Nutritional Values: Calories: 46 kcal /Carbohydrates: 3 g /Protein: 2 g /Fat: 2 g/Sodium: 28 mg

Roasted Potatoes with Rosemary and Garlic

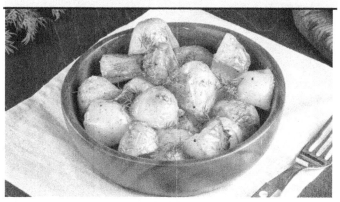

Total Time: 1 hour 10 mins / **Prep. Time:** 10 mins /**Cooking Time:** 1 hour /**Difficulty:** Easy /**Serving Size:** 4 servings

Ingredients:

- 2 large baking potatoes
- 1 tbsp. olive oil
- 2 cloves garlic, minced

- ½ tsp. crushed rosemary
- ¼ tsp. salt

Instructions:

Preheat oven to 350°F. Use a nonstick pan spray to coat a small dish or pan. Use a nonstick pan spray to coat a small dish or pan. Slice the potatoes into wedges. Arrange the potato wedges in the pan that has been prepared. In a small bowl, combine the garlic, oil, rosemary, and salt. Brush the potatoes with the oil mixture gently. Bake for 1 hour, brushing with oil every 15 minutes until soft and golden brown.

Nutritional Values: Calories: 136 kcal /Carbohydrates: 24 g /Protein: 3 g /Fat: 3 g/Sodium: 155 mg

Chapter 18: Condiments, Broths and Seasonings

Condiments are seasoning are used to add flavor and taste to the food. A condiment enhances the flavor of a food, yet it cannot be eaten on its own. It isn't a component of the dish. Instead, it is included as part of the meal to complement the main course. A sauce or gravy is an example of a condiment. No one eats sauce or gravy unless it's part of the main course.

In this chapter, you'll find several delicious and healthy Condiments, seasonings and broths persons with type-2 diabetes.

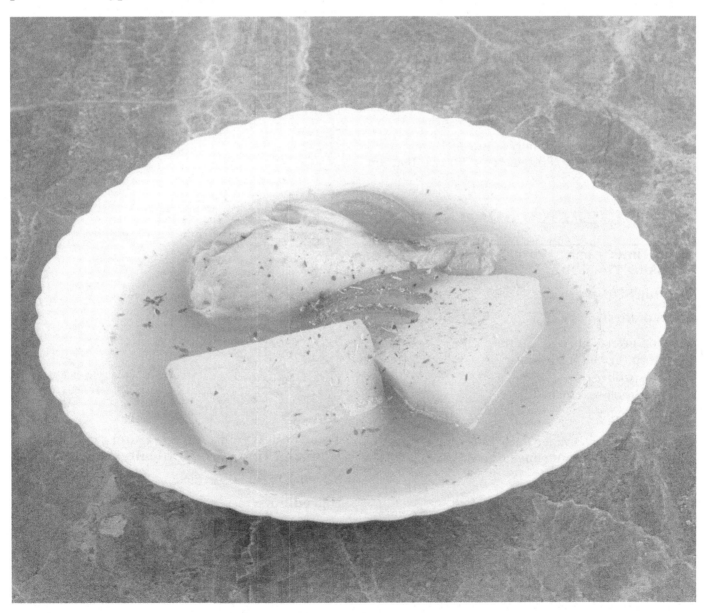

Lemon Basil Pesto

Total Time: 10 mins / **Prep. Time:** 10 mins /**Cooking Time:** N/A /**Difficulty:** Easy

Serving Size: 8 servings

Ingredients:

- 1½ cups basil leaves
- ½ tsp. grated lemon zest
- ½ cup walnuts
- 2 tbsp. soft silken tofu
- ¼ cup Asiago cheese, grated
- ½ tsp. ground black pepper
- ½ tsp. salt
- ¼ cup extra virgin olive oil

Instructions:

Pulse spinach and basil in a food processor until finely chopped. Toss in the nuts and cheese. Whirl the nuts until they're finely chopped. Toss in the tofu, salt, and pepper. Drizzle in oil while the motor is running. Toss in the lemon zest and spin to combine. Refrigerate for up to 24 hours after covering.

Nutritional Values: Calories: 140 kcal /Carbohydrates: 4 g /Protein: 3 g /Fat: 12 g/Sodium: 180 mg

Ginger-Orange Dip

Total Time: 5 mins / **Prep. Time:** 5 mins /**Cooking Time:** N/A /**Difficulty:** Easy

Serving Size: 6 servings

Ingredients:

- 3 oz. orange juice concentrate
- 1 tbsp. grated fresh ginger
- 3 tbsp. olive oil
- 1 garlic clove, crushed

Instructions:

Combine olive oil, orange juice concentrate, garlic and ginger in a medium mixing bowl. Mix thoroughly.

Nutritional Values: Calories: 15 kcal /Carbohydrates: 1 g /Protein: 0 g /Fat: 1 g/Sodium: 0 mg

Broccoli Pesto

Total Time: 10 mins / **Prep. Time:** 10 mins /**Cooking Time:** N/A /**Difficulty:** Easy

Serving Size: 8 servings

Ingredients:

- 2 cups broccoli florets
- ½ cup basil leaves, lightly packed
- 1-2 cloves garlic, chopped
- ¼ cup walnuts
- 4 tbsp. olive oil
- ¼ cup grated parmesan cheese
- black pepper grinds, to taste
- Salt, if desired

Instructions:

In a food processor or blender, combine the garlic, broccoli, basil, and nuts. Add grinds of black pepper and puree the broccoli until it is finely crushed but still has a granular texture. Drizzle in just enough oil to make the mixture creamy and soft enough to be used as dip while the machine is running. Wipe down the edges of the bowl and mix for a further 15 seconds. Place the pesto in a mixing dish. Mix in the cheese and, if preferred, season with salt. To let the flavors to mingle, cover securely and chill for 2 hours before serving.

Nutritional Values: Calories: 43 kcal /Carbohydrates: 0 g /Protein: 1 g /Fat: 4 g/Sodium: 22 mg

Creamy Garlic Dressing

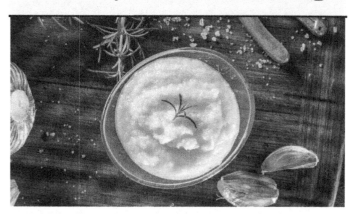

Total Time: 5 mins / **Prep. Time:** 5 mins /**Cooking Time:** N/A /**Difficulty:** Easy

Serving Size: 12 servings

Ingredients:

- ½ cup evaporated skim milk
- 2 large garlic cloves, minced
- 2 tbsp. fresh lemon juice
- 1 tsp. dried dill weed
- ¼ tsp. salt
- ¼ tsp. paprika

- 1 tsp. apple juice concentrate, frozen
- 1 tsp. sesame oil
- ¼ tsp. white pepper
- ¼ tsp. cayenne pepper

Instructions:

In a blender, combine all of the ingredients and mix until smooth.

Nutritional Values: Calories: 11 kcal /Carbohydrates: 2 g /Protein: 1 g /Fat: 0 g/Sodium: 50 mg

Cranberry-Orange Relish

Total Time: 1 hour 5 mins / **Prep. Time:** 5 mins /**Cooking Time:** 1 hour /**Difficulty:** Easy /**Serving Size:** 8 servings

Ingredients:

- 12 oz. cranberries
- 1½ cups water
- 1 orange with peel, diced
- ¼ tsp. ground cinnamon
- Sugar substitute, to taste

Instructions:

In a covered pot, simmer the orange and cranberries for 1 hour. Allow to cool before adding the sugar substitute and cinnamon. Refrigerate or freeze in 1-cup containers for up to a week.

Nutritional Values: Calories: 25 kcal /Carbohydrates: 6 g /Protein: 1 g /Fat: 0.1 g/Sodium: 9 mg

Taco Seasoning

Total Time: 5 mins / **Prep. Time:** 5 mins /**Cooking Time:** N/A /**Difficulty:** Easy

Serving Size: 1 serving

Ingredients:

- 1½ tsp. salt substitute
- 2¼ tsp. chili powder
- 1 tsp. ground cumin
- ½ tsp. onion powder
- 1 tsp. garlic powder
- ¼ tsp. ground red pepper
- 1 tsp. cornstarch

Instructions:

Combine all ingredients in a bowl. Preserve in a jar and refrigerate.

Nutritional Values: Calories: 8 kcal /Carbohydrates: 1.6 g /Protein: 0.3 g /Fat: 0 g/Sodium: 17 mg

Patty's Seasoning Blend

Total Time: 10 mins / **Prep. Time:** 5 mins /**Cooking Time:** 5 mins /**Difficulty:** Easy

Serving Size: 1 serving

Ingredients:

- 2 cloves garlic, minced
- 1 cup red or green bell pepper, chopped
- 1 1/3 cup onion, finely chopped
- 1 cup celery, chopped

Instructions:

Using cooking spray, coat a medium nonstick skillet. Cook onion, garlic, celery and bell pepper until soft, turning periodically, over medium heat. Place in a freezer bag that can be resealed. Place in the freezer until ready to use.

Nutritional Values: Calories: 26 kcal /Carbohydrates: 5.6 g /Protein: 0.8 g /Fat: 0.2 g/Sodium: 16 mg

Citrus Ginger Marinade

Total Time: 5 mins / **Prep. Time:** 5 mins /**Cooking Time:** N/A /**Difficulty:** Easy

Serving Size: 1 serving

Ingredients:

- 1 tsp. orange peel, finely grated
- 1 tsp. grated ginger
- 1 tbsp. white wine vinegar
- 3 tbsp. orange juice
- 1 tsp. olive oil

Instructions:

Combine all ingredients in a bowl. Preserve in a jar and refrigerate until ready to use.

Nutritional Values: Calories: 8.4 kcal /Carbohydrates: 0.7 g /Protein: 0 g /Fat: 0.6 g/Sodium: 0.2 mg

Bistro Dijon Sauce

Total Time: 5 mins / **Prep. Time:** 2 mins /**Cooking Time:** 3 mins /**Difficulty:** Easy

Serving Size: 1 serving

Ingredients:

- 2 tbsp. butter
- 2 cups fat-free milk
- 2 tbsp. all-purpose flour
- 2 tbsp. Dijon-style mustard

Instructions:

Melt butter in a small saucepan over medium heat. Mix in the flour well. Add the milk and continue to stir until the mixture boils. Cook it for 1 minute, or until the mixture thickens and smooths out. Remove the pan from the heat and toss in the mustard.

Nutritional Values: Calories: 29 kcal /Carbohydrates: 2.3 g /Protein: 1.2 g /Fat: 1.5 g/Sodium: 67 mg

Southwestern Lime Marinade

Total Time: 5 mins / **Prep. Time:** 5 mins /**Cooking Time:** N/A /**Difficulty:** Easy

Serving Size: 1 serving

Ingredients:

- 1 tbsp. lime juice
- 2 tbsp. olive oil
- 3 cloves garlic, peeled, halved
- 1/8 tsp. ground cumin

Instructions:

Combine all ingredients in a bowl. Preserve in a jar and refrigerate until ready to use.

Nutritional Values: Calories: 26 kcal /Carbohydrates: 0.4 g /Protein: 0.1 g /Fat: 2.7 g/Sodium: 0.2 mg

Bone Broth

Total Time: 3 hour 10 mins / **Prep. Time:** 10 mins /**Cooking Time:** 3 hours /**Difficulty:** Easy /**Serving Size:** 16 servings

Ingredients:

- 1 lb. bones of whole organic chicken
- 8 cups water
- 2 cloves garlic, minced
- 1 tsp. sea salt
- 2 tbsp. apple cider vinegar
- vegetable scraps, optional

Instructions:

In an electric pressure cooker, combine all of the ingredients. Cook for 2-3 hours on high pressure. Allow for a 10–15-minute natural pressure release before removing the lid. Remove the liquid from the strainer and place it in a container (s). It may be kept in the fridge for up to 5 days.

Nutritional Values: Calories: 60 kcal /Carbohydrates: 0.1 g /Protein: 8 g /Fat: 3 g/Sodium: 312 mg

Scotch broth

Total Time: 1 hour 10 mins / **Prep. Time:** 10 mins /**Cooking Time:** 1 hour /**Difficulty:** Easy /**Serving Size:** 4 servings

Ingredients:

- 250g stewing lamb
- 1 tbsp. olive oil
- 2 big carrots, chopped
- 200g pearl barley
- 1 leek, diced
- 1 onion, chopped
- 1 carrot, chopped
- 1 small swede, chopped
- 1 tsp. salt
- ¼ tsp. ground coriander
- ¼ tsp. white pepper
- 1 tbsp. tomato puree
- 4 cups vegetable stock
- 4 cups cold water

Instructions:

In a large sauce pan over medium heat, brown the lamb chunks in oil. Place the stewing lamb in a large skillet over high heat, cover with water, and add the vegetable stock. Combine the onion, swede, leek, carrot, and tomato puree in the pan. Rinse the barley and combine it with the salt, pepper, and powdered coriander in a pan. Cook the broth for an hour, or until the barley is mushy and the soup has thickened. Remove the lamb 20 minutes before the end of the cooking time. Allow it cool somewhat before removing the meat out from bones and discarding them. Return the lamb to the soup, cut into tiny pieces. If the soup needs extra spice or water, add it now and serve.

Nutritional Values: Calories: 621 kcal /Carbohydrates: 20 g /Protein: 57 g /Fat: 13 g/Sodium: 630 mg

Vegetable Broth

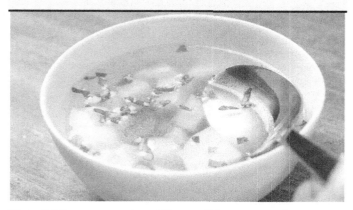

Total Time: 35 mins / **Prep. Time:** 10 mins /**Cooking Time:** 25 mins /**Difficulty:** Easy /**Serving Size:** 6 servings

Ingredients:

- 6 cups water
- 1 onion, chopped
- 1 tbsp. canola oil
- 3 cloves garlic, crushed
- 1 carrot, chopped
- 2 bay leaves
- 2 stalks celery, chopped
- ½ tsp. salt
- 5 sprigs parsley

Instructions:

In a normal saucepan, heat the canola oil. Sauté vegetables for 5 minutes or until onion, garlic, carrot, and celery are aromatic. Bring the remaining ingredients to a boil. Reduce heat to low and cook for 25 minutes. Remove from heat and set aside to cool. When the stock has cooled, drain it, carefully pushing the liquid out of the veggies for more flavors. Vegetables should be discarded.

Nutritional Values: Calories: 32 kcal /Carbohydrates: 3 g /Protein: 0 g /Fat: 2 g/Sodium: 87 mg

Mixed Bones Broth

Total Time: 5 hour 10 mins / **Prep. Time:** 10 mins /**Cooking Time:** 5 hours /**Difficulty:** Easy /**Serving Size:** 4 servings

Ingredients:

- 1 lb. mixed bones (chicken, beef, lamb, pork, etc.)
- 4 cups cold water

Instructions:

Preheat the oven to 400°F. Place the bones on a parchment paper or foil-lined sheet tray. Roast bones for 45 minutes to 1 hour, or until dark brown. Place the roasted bones in a saucepan with care. Fill the pan with cold water up the level of the bones, but not higher. The top of the pot's bones should just be slightly submerged. Place the saucepan over medium heat and gently bring to a boil, then reduce to the lowest possible simmer. You simply need to glimpse a bubble now and then. Cook for 4 hours. Using cheesecloth or sieves, strain the liquid. Allow it cool for an hour or two on the counter before placing in the refrigerator.

Nutritional Values: Calories: 45 kcal /Carbohydrates: 5 g /Protein: 20 g /Fat: 0.5 g/Sodium: 10 mg

Lamb Broth

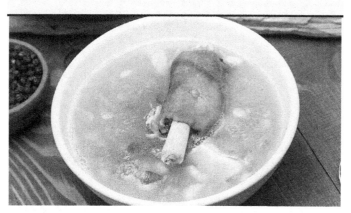

Total Time: 2 hour 30 mins / **Prep. Time:** 30 mins /**Cooking Time:** 2 hours /**Difficulty:** Easy /**Serving Size:** 4 servings

Ingredients:

- 1½ lb. lamb bones
- 1 carrot, peeled
- 1 onion, peeled
- ½ cup parsley stems
- ½ cup celery leaves
- 1 tsp. salt
- 1 clove garlic, peeled
- 8 whole black peppercorns

Instructions:

In a stockpot, place the lamb bones. Add 12 cups cold water, or enough to cover the bottom of the pan Bring to a boil, and then skim the foam away. Add the other ingredients and cook for 2 hours on low heat, slightly covered. Remove the bone and vegetables from the broth and strain it through a fine strainer. Allow to cool. Allow to cool before skimming off the fat.

Nutritional Values: Calories: 21 kcal
/Carbohydrates: 5 g /Protein: 0.1 g /Fat: 0.7
g/Sodium: 597 mg

Chapter 19: Dessert Recipes

Just because you are diagnosed with type 2 diabetes doesn't imply, you'll never be able to eat anything sweet again. There are methods to fulfil your cravings from time - to - time with a little planning.

If you have diabetes, as per the American Diabetes Association, you can consume sweets and desserts if they're part of a balanced eating plan and you don't overindulge.

In this chapter, you'll find several healthy and delicious desserts recipe for people with type-2 diabetes.

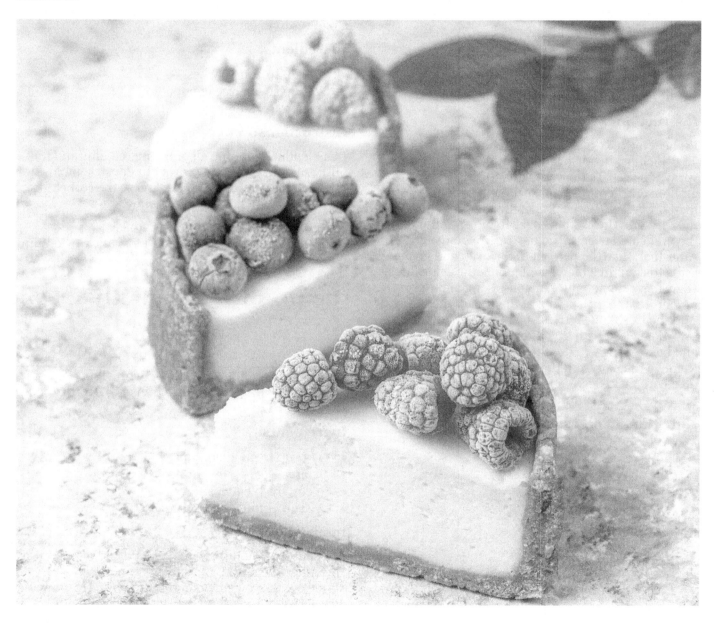

Blueberry Yogurt Lemon Bars

Total Time: 55 mins / **Prep. Time:** 10 mins /**Cooking Time:** 45 mins /**Difficulty:** Medium/**Serving Size:** 16 servings

Ingredients:

- Nonstick cooking spray
- 1 1/2 cup graham cracker flour, unsweetened
- 2 tsp + 1 tbsp. lemon zest, divided
- ¼ tsp. fine sea salt
- 3 tbsp. avocado oil
- 3 egg whites
- 1 whole egg
- 1 tsp. maple syrup
- ¾ cup fresh blueberries
- 2 cup nonfat vanilla Greek yogurt
- ¼ cup lemon juice, freshly squeezed

Instructions:

Preheat oven to 350 °F. Use parchment paper to line an 8-inch baking dish, and then spray it with cooking spray. To prepare the crust, mix together avocado oil, graham cracker flour, 2 tbsp. lemon zest, and salt in a food processor. In the prepared pan, press the mixture into the bottom. Bake for 10–15 minutes in the preheated oven till golden brown on the crust. After that, take the pan out of the oven and lay it aside to cool. In a blender, combine the egg whites, yogurt, egg, lemon juice, maple syrup, and the remaining 1 tbsp. lemon zest to prepare the filling. Add the fresh blueberries and mix well. Fill the prebaked crust with the filling. Preheat oven to 350°F and bake for 25–30 minutes, till the centre is set. Remove the pan from the oven and cool thoroughly on a wire rack. Serve refrigerated or at room temperature, cut into 16 equal-sized squares.

Nutritional Values: Calories: 90 kcal /Carbohydrates: 10 g /Protein: 4 g /Fat: 4 g/Sodium: 105 mg

Pineapple Peach Sorbet

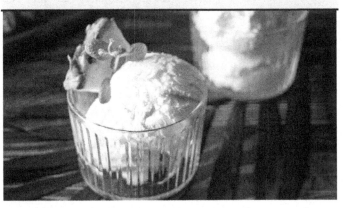

Total Time: 4 hour 5 mins / **Prep. Time:** 5 mins /**Cooking Time:** N/A /**Difficulty:** Easy /**Serving Size:** 2 servings

Ingredients:

- ½ cup frozen peaches
- ¼ cup sugar-free lemonade
- ½ cup frozen pineapple chunks

Instructions:

In a blender, combine all of the ingredients and mix until smooth. Freeze the sorbet in Popsicle molds or a container as soon as possible. Freeze the sorbet for 4 hours or overnight. Serve and enjoy.

Nutritional Values: Calories: 40 kcal /Carbohydrates: 10 g /Protein: 1 g /Fat: 0 g/Sodium: 0 mg

Lemon Chiffon with Fresh Berries

Total Time: 1 hour 20 mins / **Prep. Time:** 1 hour 10 mins /**Cooking Time:** 10 mins /**Difficulty:** Easy /**Serving Size:** 6 servings

Ingredients:

- 1/3 cup fresh lemon juice
- 4 large eggs
- 3 cup fresh berries
- ½ cup granulated Splenda

Instructions:

In a saucepan, combine the Splenda and lemon juice. Heat and whisk until the sugar is completely dissolved. Remove the pan from the heat. In a mixing dish, crack the eggs and whisk them thoroughly. While stirring, slowly add the lemon sugar mixture into the eggs. Return the egg mix to the pot after 1 minute of whisking. Cook for several minutes over low to medium heat, whisking constantly, until the egg mixture thickens. Depending on your equipment, this will take 2-5 minutes. When the mixture coats the back of a spoon, it's time to take it off the heat. Refrigerate for at least one hour. As it cools, it will thicken even more. Spoon berries over some of the lemon chiffon in a dessert dish or glass, or stack lemon cream and berries. Garnish with berries.

Nutritional Values: Calories: 90 kcal /Carbohydrates: 11 g /Protein: 5 g /Fat: 3 g/Sodium: 50 mg

Berry Crisp

Total Time: 1 hour 10 mins / **Prep. Time:** 15 mins /**Cooking Time:** 55 mins /**Difficulty:** Medium/**Serving Size:** 8 servings

Ingredients:

- 1 nonstick cooking spray
- 1 pint blueberries
- 1 tsp. lemon zest
- 1 lb. Strawberries, sliced
- 3 tbsp. Splenda Sugar Blend
- 1½ tbsp. corn starch
- 2 tbsp. lemon juice
- 1 tsp. ground cinnamon
- 3 tbsp. Brown Sugar Blend
- ½ cup pecans, chopped
- 1 cup old-fashioned rolled oats
- 4 tbsp. trans-fat-free margarine, cubed

Instructions:

Preheat oven to 350 °F. Using cooking spray, coat a 9-inch pie tin. Combine the lemon zest, corn starch, berries, 2 tbsp. Splenda sugar blend and 2 tbsp. lemon juice in a medium mixing bowl. Combine all ingredients and pour into a pie plate. Combine the oats, brown sugar blend, remaining 1 tbsp. Splenda sugar blend, pecans, and margarine in a medium mixing bowl. Working with your hands, crumble the margarine into the dry ingredients. Over the berries, evenly distribute the crisp topping mixture. Bake for 55 minutes, or until the fruit is bubbling and the top is golden. Serve warm and enjoy.

Nutritional Values: Calories: 190 kcal /Carbohydrates: 24 g /Protein: 3 g /Fat: 11 g/Sodium: 50 mg

Pumpkin-Vanilla Pudding

Total Time: 17 mins / **Prep. Time:** 10 mins /**Cooking Time:** 7 mins /**Difficulty:** Easy /**Serving Size:** 8 servings

Ingredients:

- 1 whipped topping
- 1 vanilla bean
- ¼ cup pecans
- ¼ tsp. ground ginger
- 1/8 tsp. ground nutmeg
- ¼ tsp. ground cloves
- 8 oz. canned pumpkin
- 1 tsp. ground cinnamon
- 2 eggs
- 2 tbsp. corn starch
- 1¾ cup 1% milk
- ¼ cup Splenda sugar blend

Instructions:

Whisk together the corn starch and sweetener in a 3-quart pot. Whisk together the egg yolks and milk in a small bowl. Gradually whisk the sweetener mixture into the egg mixture over medium heat. Bring to a boil, whisking constantly until the mixture thickens, approximately 3 to 5 minutes. Combine the pumpkin, cloves, cinnamon, nutmeg and ginger in a mixing bowl. Cook for 3 minutes on low heat after thoroughly mixing. Cook for another minute after adding the vanilla bean seeds. Take the pot off the heat. Wrap the pudding with plastic wrap and place it in a bowl. Before serving, chill for 1 hour. To serve, pour the pudding into individual dessert glasses, top with 1/2 tablespoon nuts, and sprinkle with cinnamon. Dollop with whipped topping and enjoy.

Nutritional Values: Calories: 85 kcal /Carbohydrates: 9 g /Protein: 3 g /Fat: 4 g/Sodium: 30 mg

Mini-Pumpkin Tarts

Total Time: 40 mins / **Prep. Time:** 10 mins /**Cooking Time:** 30 mins /**Difficulty:** Easy /**Serving Size:** 30 servings

Ingredients:

- 8 oz. light cream cheese, softened
- ¼ cup light sour cream
- 30 wafer cookies
- 1 egg
- ¼ cup Splenda sugar blend
- ½ tsp. vanilla extract

- ½ tsp. ground cinnamon
- ¾ cup canned pure pumpkin
- 1 pinch ground nutmeg

Instructions:

Lay one wafer in the bottom of every cup in a mini-muffin pan lined with paper baking cups. Add the remaining ingredients to a medium mixing bowl and beat with an electric mixer until smooth. Pour the pumpkin-cream cheese mixture into each muffin cup. Preheat the oven to 350°F and bake the muffins for 30 minutes, or until done. Allow to cool before serving.

Nutritional Values: Calories: 40 kcal /Carbohydrates: 4 g /Protein: 1 g /Fat: 2 g/Sodium: 40 mg

Chia Seed Falooda

Total Time: 8 hour 20 mins / **Prep. Time:** 8 hour 10 mins /**Cooking Time:** N/A /**Difficulty:** Easy

Serving Size: 8 servings

Ingredients:

- ½ cup chia seeds
- 1 tsp. vanilla extract
- 2½ cup low fat milk
- ½ cup raspberries
- 2 tsp. rose water
- ¼ cup cooked soba noodles
- 1 tbsp. maple syrup
- 1½ tbsp. lemon juice
- ½ cup pomegranate seeds

Instructions:

Combine milk and chia seeds in a large mixing bowl. Chia seeds should be soaked for minimum 8 hours or overnight in the fridge. Add vanilla extract once the chia seeds have soaked. Set aside after thoroughly mixing. Combine the maple syrup, raspberries, lemon and rose water in a medium mixing bowl. Set aside after gently stirring to blend. Put a thin layer of raspberry sauce, a layer of chia seed mixture, and a thin layer of soba noodles in a short glass. Repeat for each dish, finishing with pomegranate seeds on top.

Nutritional Values: Calories: 120 kcal /Carbohydrates: 15 g /Protein: 5 g /Fat: 5 g/Sodium: 40 mg

Fig and Walnut Yogurt Tarts

Total Time: 15 mins / **Prep. Time:** 15 mins /**Cooking Time:** N/A /**Difficulty:** Easy

Serving Size: 6 servings

Ingredients:

- 1 oz. crumbled goat cheese
- ¼ cup nonfat, plain Greek yogurt
- 2 tbsp. freshly squeezed orange juice
- 12 mini phyllo dough shells
- 12 leaves fresh mint, chopped
- 12 walnut halves
- 4 large fresh figs, chopped

Instructions:

Combine yogurt, goat cheese and orange juice in a small mixing bowl. Fill 1 tbsp. of the cheese mixture into each phyllo shell. Place a walnut half, 1 mint leaf, and a fig slice on top of each. Keep it refrigerated before serving and enjoy.

Nutritional Values: Calories: 130 kcal /Carbohydrates: 14 g /Protein: 4 g /Fat: 7 g/Sodium: 60 mg

Peanut Butter Cookies

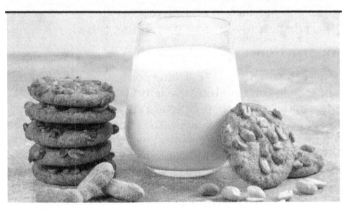

Total Time: 20 mins / **Prep. Time:** 20 mins /**Cooking Time:** 10 mins /**Difficulty:** Easy /**Serving Size:** 20 servings

Ingredients:

- 1 cup peanut butter
- 1 large egg, beaten
- 1 tsp. vanilla extract
- 1 cup Splenda granulated sweetener

Instructions:

Combine Splenda sweetener, peanut butter, vanilla extract and egg in a large mixing bowl. Refrigerate the mixture for at least ten minutes. Make 1 tablespoon balls with the ingredients and arrange them on an ungreased sheet pan. To make a crosshatch design, lightly press each biscuit with the tines of a fork and flatten slightly. Preheat oven to 350°F and bake for 8 minutes. Allow to cool for at least 5 minutes on the sheet pan before moving to a wire rack to complete cooling.

Nutritional Values: Calories: 80 kcal /Carbohydrates: 3 g /Protein: 4 g /Fat: 7 g/Sodium: 50 mg

Banana Chocolate Ice Cream

Total Time: 2 hour 30 mins / **Prep. Time:** 2 hour 30 mins /**Cooking Time:** N/A /**Difficulty:** Easy /**Serving Size:** 5 servings

Ingredients:

- 2 medium bananas
- 2 tbsp. cocoa powder
- 1 cup whipped topping, fat-free
- 1/3 cup skim milk

Instructions:

Bananas should be peeled and sliced into quarter-inch coins. Freeze the sliced bananas for at least 2 hours after placing in a bowl. Once the bananas are frozen, combine them with the milk and chocolate powder. Blend until completely smooth. Fold in the whipped topping until it is evenly distributed. Freeze the mixture for at least 30 minutes in a freezer-safe container. To serve, scoop into 1/2-cup scoops and enjoy.

Nutritional Values: Calories: 80 kcal /Carbohydrates: 18 g /Protein: 2 g /Fat: 0.5 g/Sodium: 15 mg

Pineapple Fluff

Total Time: 10 mins + Chilling / **Prep. Time:** 10 mins /**Cooking Time:** N/A /**Difficulty:** Easy /**Serving Size:** 8 servings

Ingredients:

- 1 package instant vanilla pudding mix, sugar free
- 12 oz. low-fat whipped topping, divided

- 15 oz. pineapple with juice

Instructions:

Combine the pineapple juice and pudding mix in a medium mixing bowl. Fold in one-third of the whipped topping at a time, softly mixing after each addition. Fill 8 dessert bowls with the mixture. Refrigerate until the pudding has firmed up.

Nutritional Values: Calories: 137 kcal /Carbohydrates: 21 g /Protein: 1.5 g /Fat: 5.6 g/Sodium: 144 mg

Chocolate Pudding

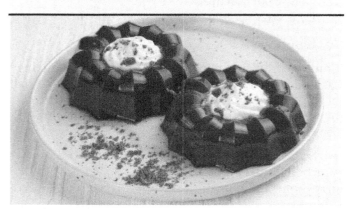

Total Time: 20 mins + chilling / **Prep. Time:** 5 mins /**Cooking Time:** 15 mins /**Difficulty:** Easy /**Serving Size:** 6 servings

Ingredients:

- 1/3 cup Splenda sugar blend
- 2 tbsp. cornstarch
- ¼ cup unsweetened cocoa
- ¼ cups reduced-fat milk
- 1/8 tsp. salt
- 1 tsp. vanilla extract

Instructions:

Combine the cocoa, cornstarch, Splenda sugar blend, and salt in a medium saucepan. Stir in the milk gradually. Cook, stirring regularly, over medium heat until the mixture boils. Remove from the heat and mix in the vanilla extract. Refrigerate for 2 to 3 hours, or until firm, in 6 individual serving plates or 1 big bowl.

Nutritional Values: Calories: 119 kcal /Carbohydrates: 20 g /Protein: 3.7 g /Fat: 2.3 g/Sodium: 93 mg

Berry-Berry Pudding Surprise

Total Time: 5 mins / **Prep. Time:** 5 mins /**Cooking Time:** N/A /**Difficulty:** Easy

Serving Size: 10 servings

Ingredients:

- 2 packages instant white chocolate pudding mix, sugar-free
- 4 cups sliced fresh strawberries
- 4 cups fat-free milk
- 8 oz. fat-free whipped topping

Instructions:

Combine milk and pudding mix in a medium mixing dish and stir well. Spread half of the pudding and half of the strawberry slices in a trifle dish or big glass bowl. Layers should be repeated. Serve with whipped topping on top.

Nutritional Values: Calories: 112 kcal /Carbohydrates: 21 g /Protein: 5.2 g /Fat: 1.4 g/Sodium: 146 mg

Coconut Pudding

Total Time: 5 mins + chilling / **Prep. Time:** 5 mins /**Cooking Time:** N/A /**Difficulty:** Easy /**Serving Size:** 4 servings

Ingredients:

- 2 cups fat-free milk
- ¼ tsp. coconut extract
- 1 package instant vanilla pudding mix, sugar-free
- 2 tbsp. shredded coconut, toasted

Instructions:

Combine pudding mix, milk, and coconut extract in a blender and process for about 1 minute, or until slightly thickened. Sprinkle with coconut and divide among 4 dessert bowls. Refrigerate for 30 minutes, or until completely set.

Nutritional Values: Calories: 84 kcal /Carbohydrates: 14 g /Protein: 4.2 g /Fat: 1.1 g/Sodium: 397 mg

Chocolate Almond Pudding

Total Time: 20 mins + chilling / **Prep. Time:** 5 mins /**Cooking Time:** 15 mins /**Difficulty:** Easy /**Serving Size:** 6 servings

Ingredients:

- 1/3 cup Splenda sugar blend
- 2 tbsp. cornstarch
- ¼ cup unsweetened cocoa
- 2¼ cups reduced fat milk
- 1/8 tsp. salt
- ½ cup fat-free whipped topping
- 1 tsp. almond extract
- 1 tsp. sliced almonds

Instructions:

Combine cocoa, Splenda sugar blend, salt and cornstarch in a medium saucepan. Stir in the milk gradually. Cook, stirring regularly, over medium heat until the mixture boils. Remove the pan from the heat and add the almond extract. Refrigerate for 2 to 3 hours, or until set, in 6 individual serving plates or 1 big bowl. Add a dollop of whipped topping and a sprinkling of almonds on top.

Nutritional Values: Calories: 108 kcal /Carbohydrates: 19 g /Protein: 3.6 g /Fat: 0.7 g/Sodium: 102 mg

Peanut Butter Cookies

Total Time: 20 mins / **Prep. Time:** 5 mins /**Cooking Time:** 15 mins /**Difficulty:** Easy /**Serving Size:** 12 servings

Ingredients:

- 1 cup smooth peanut butter, without sugar
- 2/3 cup erythritol
- 1 large egg
- ½ tsp. vanilla essence
- ½ tsp. baking soda

Instructions:

Preheat the oven to 350°F and line a cookie sheet with parchment paper. In a blender, mix the erythritol until it is powdered. In a medium mixing bowl, combine all of the ingredients and stir until a smooth, shiny dough forms. To make a ball, roll roughly 2 tablespoons of dough between your palms and place on the prepared cookie pan. Continue until all the dough has been utilized. You should have 12-

14 cookies at the end. Flatten the cookies with a fork, making a crisscross pattern over the top. Preheat the oven to 350°F and bake the cookies for 15 minutes.

Nutritional Values: Calories: 140 kcal /Carbohydrates: 4 g /Protein: 6 g /Fat: 10 g/Sodium: 134 mg

Chocolate Bombs

Total Time: 15 mins + chilling / **Prep. Time:** 15 mins /**Cooking Time:** N/A /**Difficulty:** Easy /**Serving Size:** 12 servings

Ingredients:

- 2 tbsp. heavy cream
- 1 tsp. vanilla extract
- ¼ cup unsweetened Cacao powder
- 6 tbsp. hemp seeds (shelled)
- ½ cup unrefined coconut oil
- 5 tbsp. natural chunky peanut butter
- 2 tbsp. Stevia

Instructions:

In a large mixing dish, combine peanut butter, cocoa powder, and hemp seeds. Mix in the room temperature coconut oil until it forms a paste. Mix in the vanilla, cream, and stevia until the mixture resembles a paste. Make balls out of the dough. In all, you should be able to manufacture roughly 12 balls. If the paste is too runny to roll, chill it for 30 minutes before attempting to do so. Place the balls on a baking pan lined with parchment paper. Before serving, freeze for 10 minutes or chill for at least 30 minutes.

Nutritional Values: Calories: 194 kcal /Carbohydrates: 3 g /Protein: 17 g /Fat: 4 g/Sodium: 1 mg

Protein Cheesecake

Total Time: 1 hour / **Prep. Time:** 10 mins /**Cooking Time:** 50 mins /**Difficulty:** Medium/**Serving Size:** 2 servings

Ingredients:

- 8.5 oz. low fat cottage cheese
- 1 scoop vanilla protein powder
- 1 tbsp. Stevia
- 2 egg whites
- 1 serving sugar-free Strawberry Jell-O
- 1 tsp. vanilla extract
- Water

Instructions:

Preheat the oven to 325°F. Place the Jell-O in the freezer after following the packaging directions. Combine egg whites and cottage cheese in a blender until smooth. In a mixing dish, combine the combined mixture with the Stevia, protein powder, and vanilla extract. Bake for 25 minutes on a small nonstick pan with the batter. Turn the oven off but leave the cake in there to cool. Remove the cheesecake from the oven after it has cooled. Pour the Jell-O over the cheesecake when it's almost set. Allow at least 10-12 hours for the cake to set in the refrigerator before serving.

Nutritional Values: Calories: 165 kcal /Carbohydrates: 6 g /Protein: 32 g /Fat: 1 g/Sodium: 560 mg

Chocolate Greek Yogurt Ice Cream

Total Time: 5 mins + chilling / **Prep. Time:** 5 mins /**Cooking Time:** N/A /**Difficulty:** Easy /**Serving Size:** 1 serving

Ingredients:

- 2½ oz. fat-free Greek yogurt
- 1 tsp. unsweetened cocoa powder
- ½ cup unsweetened almond milk
- ½ oz. vanilla protein powder
- 2 tbsp. Stevia to taste
- 1 tsp. vanilla extract
- Almonds & berries, optional

Instructions:

Completely combine the yoghurt, protein powder, stevia, chocolate, and almond milk in a blender. Place in the freezer or in an ice cream maker. If creating ice cream in the freezer, take it out after an hour and gently flip it over with a spoon to prevent it from forming one large ice block. Repeat this process every 30 minutes until the ice cream has reached the desired consistency.

Nutritional Values: Calories: 127 kcal /Carbohydrates: 8 g /Protein: 20 g /Fat: 2 g/Sodium: 150 mg

Raspberry and Banana Mousse

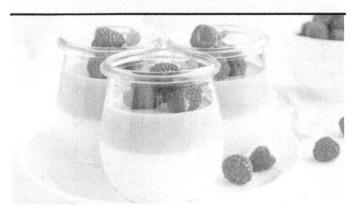

Total Time: 5 mins / **Prep. Time:** 5 mins /**Cooking Time:** N/A /**Difficulty:** Easy

Serving Size: 1 serving

Ingredients:

- 2 egg whites
- 2 oz. frozen banana
- 1 tbsp. Stevia
- Fresh berries, optional
- ¾ oz. frozen raspberry

Instructions:

Blend the egg whites with the Stevia until they are stiff. The egg whites should not fall out of the blender if you hold it upside down. Add the berries and banana when the egg whites are set. Blend until everything is pink and the consistency is silky. Serve with some few fresh berries in a dish.

Nutritional Values: Calories: 122 kcal /Carbohydrates: 11 g /Protein: 19 g /Fat: 0 g/Sodium: 153 mg

COOKING CONVERSION CHART

Measurement

CUP	ONCES	MILLILITERS	TABLESPOONS
8 cup	64 oz	1895 ml	128
6 cup	48 oz	1420 ml	96
5 cup	40 oz	1180 ml	80
4 cup	32 oz	960 ml	64
2 cup	16 oz	480 ml	32
1 cup	8 oz	240 ml	16
3/4 cup	6 oz	177 ml	12
2/3 cup	5 oz	158 ml	11
1/2 cup	4 oz	118 ml	8
3/8 cup	3 oz	90 ml	6
1/3 cup	2.5 oz	79 ml	5.5
1/4 cup	2 oz	59 ml	4
1/8 cup	1 oz	30 ml	3
1/16 cup	1/2 oz	15 ml	1

Temperature

FAHRENHEIT	CELSIUS
100 °F	37 °C
150 °F	65 °C
200 °F	93 °C
250 °F	121 °C
300 °F	150 °C
325 °F	160 °C
350 °F	180 °C
375 °F	190 °C
400 °F	200 °C
425 °F	220 °C
450 °F	230 °C
500 °F	260 °C
525 °F	274 °C
550 °F	288 °C

Weight

IMPERIAL	METRIC
1/2 oz	15 g
1 oz	29 g
2 oz	57 g
3 oz	85 g
4 oz	113 g
5 oz	141 g
6 oz	170 g
8 oz	227 g
10 oz	283 g
12 oz	340 g
13 oz	369 g
14 oz	397 g
15 oz	425 g
1 lb	453 g

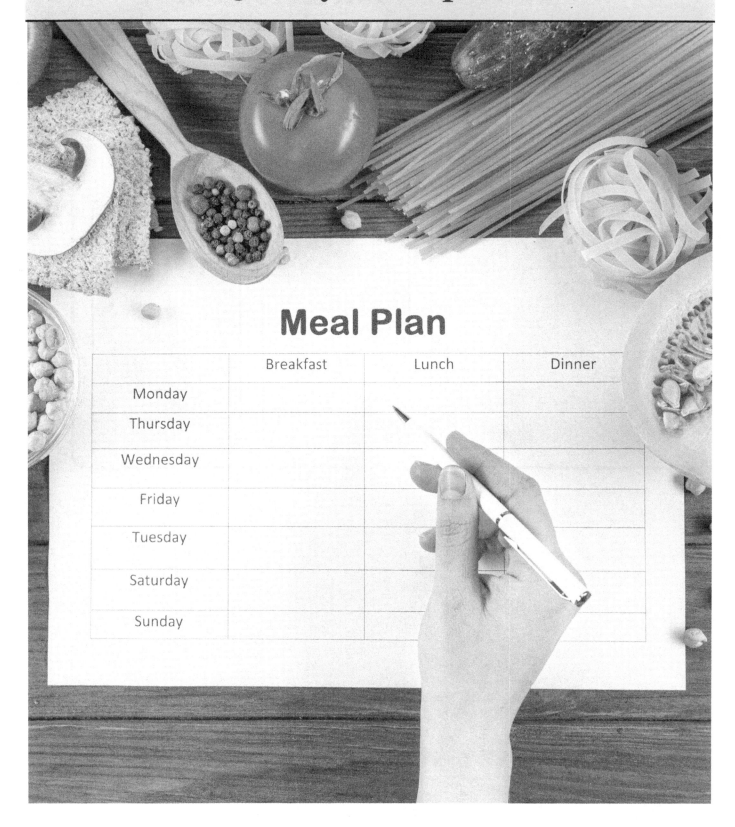

Meal Plan

	Breakfast	Lunch	Dinner
Monday			
Thursday			
Wednesday			
Friday			
Tuesday			
Saturday			
Sunday			

Days	Breakfast	Lunch	Dinner
1	Yogurt Pancakes	Skillet Chicken Tenders	Sweet and Tangy Salmon
2	Quinoa Breakfast Bowl	Chicken Philly Cheesesteak	Peppered Tuna Kabobs
3	Whole Grain Banana Pancakes	Hamburger Vegetable Soup	Zucchini Lasagna
4	Hawaiian Hash	Tomato Pie	Stuffed Chicken Breast
5	Classic Avocado Toast	Turkey Roll-Up	Cajun Beef and Rice
6	Buttermilk Pumpkin Waffles	Rotisserie Chicken	Cheesy Crispy Diabetic Pizza
7	Southwest Breakfast Wraps	Pork Tacos With Mango Salsa	Chicken Ricotta
8	Vegetarian Lentils With Egg Toast	Chicken With Peach-Avocado Salsa	Beef and Veggie Chili
9	Cinnamon Chia Seed Pudding	Chicken And Spanish Cauliflower Rice	Italian Beef and Cheese Bowl
10	Apple Pie Oats	Grilled Chicken Chopped Salad	Cabbage and Meat Gravy
11	Cauliflower Cups	Fish Tacos	Greek Yogurt Chicken
12	Spanish Omelette	Sesame Chicken with Couscous	Pork Chops with Mexican Rice
13	Raspberry Chia Pudding	Grilled Chicken and Greens	Quick and Easy Vegetable Curry
14	Breakfast Egg Muffins	Sesame Turkey Stir-Fry	Hawaiian Chicken Packets
15	Vegetable Frittata	Summer Garden Fish Tacos	Cinnamon Chicken
16	Cranberry Orange Scones	Shrimp Orzo with Feta	Grilled Rosemary Chicken
17	Flourless Banana Pancakes	Garlic Tilapia	Orange-Glazed Pork

			Chops
18	Crunchy Blueberry Yoghurt	Healthy Tuscan Chicken	Lemon Caper Tilapia
19	Traditional Porridge	Spicy Turkey Tenderloin	Orange Chicken
20	Parmesan Herb Frittata	Artichoke Ratatouille Chicken	Basil Grilled Shrimp
21	Apple Spiced Overnight Oats	Lemon-Lime Salmon	Herb Marinated Chicken
22	Fruity Nutty Muesli	Savory Pork Salad	Sun-Dried Tomato Salmon
23	Brussels Sprouts Casserole	Cobb Salad Wraps	Simple Beef Stir-Fry
24	Almond Flour Pancakes	Pork Grapefruit Stir-Fry	Herb-Grilled Bass
25	Cauliflower Fritters	Spicy Coconut Shrimp with Quinoa	Apricot Glazed Chicken
26	Cottage Cheese Breakfast Bowl	Zippy Turkey Zoodles	Steak and Portobello Sandwich
27	Raspberry Chia Pudding	Tuscan Fish Packets	Teriyaki Chicken
28	Spanish Omelette	Italian Chicken	Simple Grilled Salmon
29	Apple Pie Oats	Veggie and Hummus Sandwich	Rosemary Chicken
30	Cranberry Muffins	Quesadillas	Braised Herbed Chicken

Conclusion

Every day, you make eating decisions. Which is better: whole wheat or white bread? Fresh fruits or a plate of French fries? Do you want to eat now or later?

One of the most important aspects of diabetes control is your nutrition. Palinski-Wade explains that "what you consume might assist or hinder insulin resistance." Your blood sugar (glucose), as well as your blood pressure and cholesterol, are affected by the foods you consume, when you eat them, and how much of them you eat. The first step in controlling diabetes is to understand how diet influences blood glucose levels. Whatever diet or eating pattern you pick, make sure to consume a wide range of nutrient-dense foods and keep track of your portions.

Eat meals that are dense with nutrients and are based on combination of complex carbohydrates, proteins, and healthy fats and follow a diabetes meal plan can also help you stay on track with your blood glucose levels.

Made in the USA
Coppell, TX
01 October 2022

83875317R00096